Sleeping Better in Pregnancy

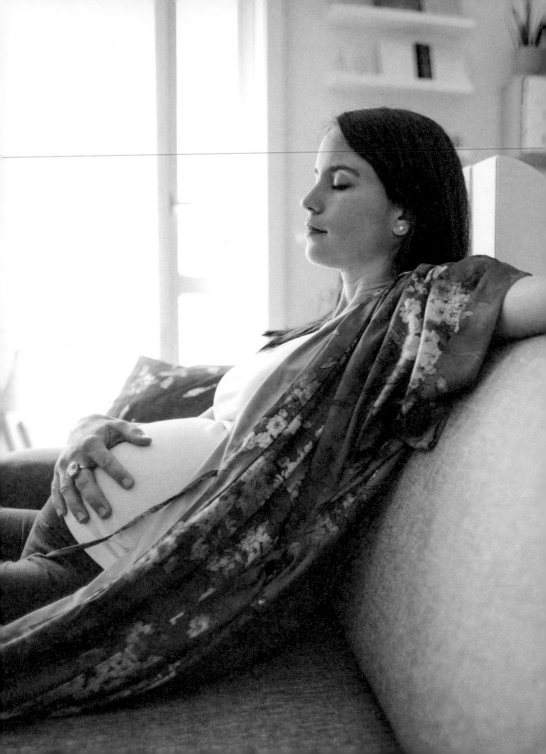

Sleeping Better in Pregnancy

A GUIDE TO SLEEP HEALTH

CLARE LADYMAN
with Leigh Signal
SLEEP/WAKE RESEARCH CENTRE

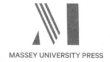

MASSEY UNIVERSITY PRESS

Contents

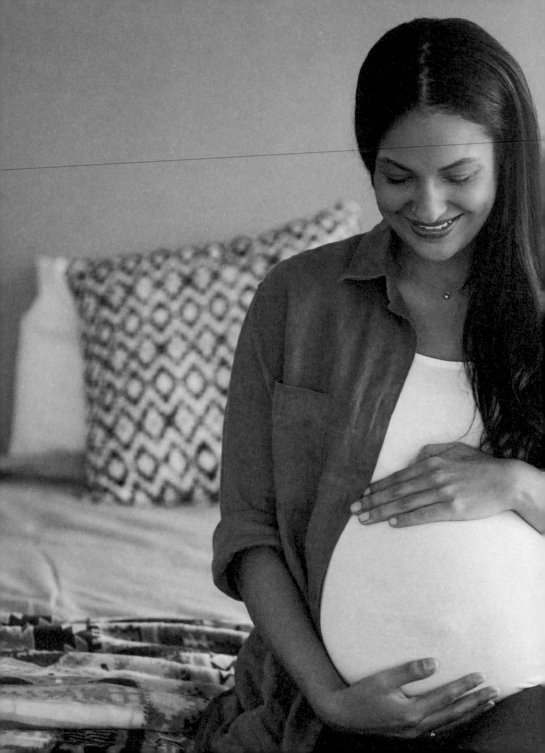

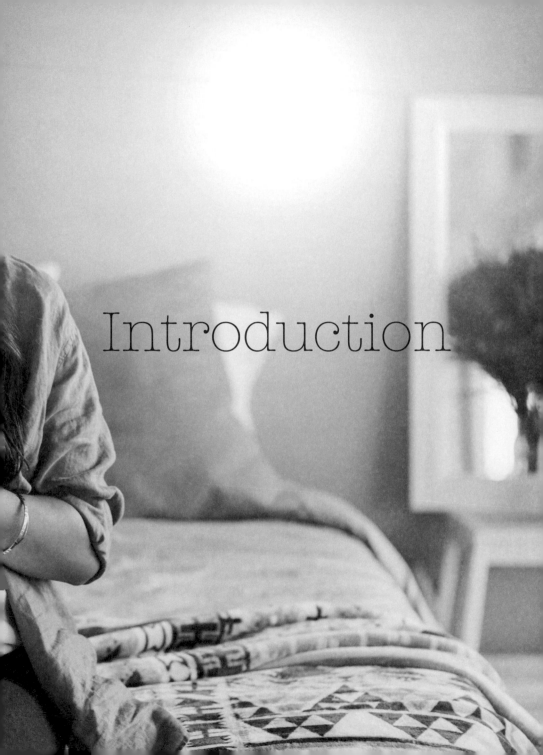

Introduction

It's a weird feeling. I know things are going to change, but I don't know how they're going to change. Even with all the information out there, it's all so new.

— HOLLY (31)

Having a baby is one of life's most amazing events. While being pregnant is a special time, it's also a time of enormous change. Your body is changing quickly and you may find you are thinking and sleeping differently, too. You may be experiencing a dozen different emotions on a daily or even an hourly basis: you may be feeling uncertain or anxious, excited or relaxed. Pregnancy is different for everyone, and how your body and mind adjust is unique to you.

Your healthcare provider, pregnancy books and trusted websites can guide you through what is happening to your body, how your baby is growing, what you should eat, how you should exercise. But it is difficult to get helpful, accurate information on sleep in pregnancy. This is mainly because sleep health research is a relatively new topic. Only recently have we become aware of how much sleep affects every aspect of our physical and mental wellbeing.

Research on sleep health in pregnancy is an even newer field, probably because there has been so much focus on mothers' sleep once the baby has arrived. Recent research has shown how crucial it is to get healthy sleep while pregnant, but this can be difficult. The huge changes in your body impact your sleep, and nearly all women will experience sleep disruption of some kind. But if you are able to manage your sleep well over the next few months, the immediate and long-term benefits for both you and your baby can be substantial.

That's how we want to help you with this book. We'll give you the most current information on sleep changes you can expect while pregnant. Being prepared for a range of possibilities can help you develop realistic expectations about your sleep in the next few months. There will be some challenges in meeting your sleep needs while your body is busy growing your baby, but the ideas and information in the following pages will hopefully assist you in making the most of your sleep opportunities, so you can stay well and enjoy this special time.

This book is divided into five sections. The first section describes why sleep is important and how it works. The second section explains some overall sleep strategies to help you with your sleep throughout pregnancy; and the next three sections look at sleep strategies during the three trimesters of pregnancy. You might notice that there is some repetition in these trimester sections. This is because some sleep changes occur in more than one trimester, and other changes are more trimester-specific. This repetition is intentional so that you can pick the book up at any time in your pregnancy and read about the sleep for that trimester.

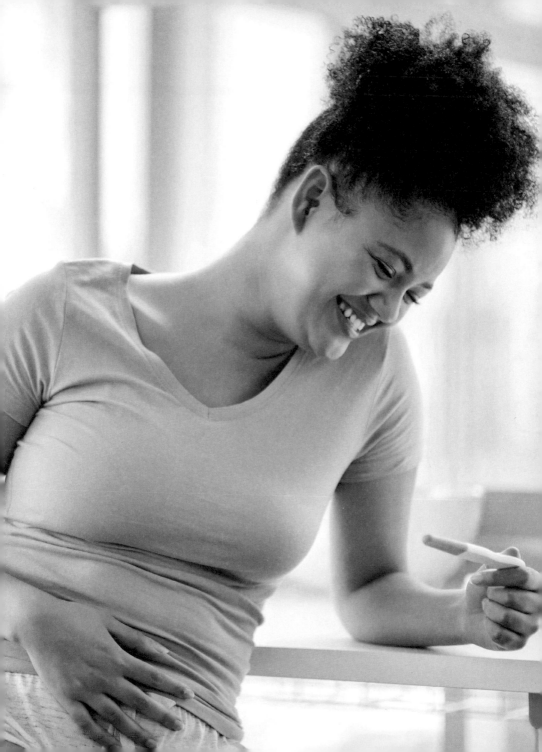

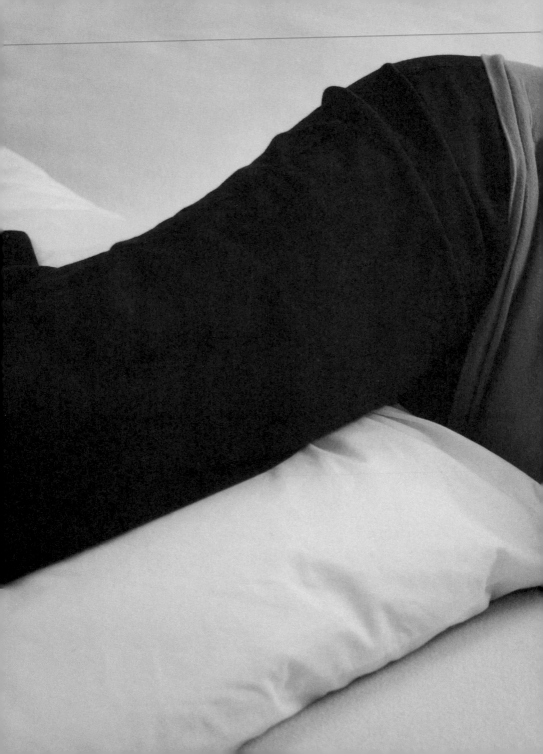

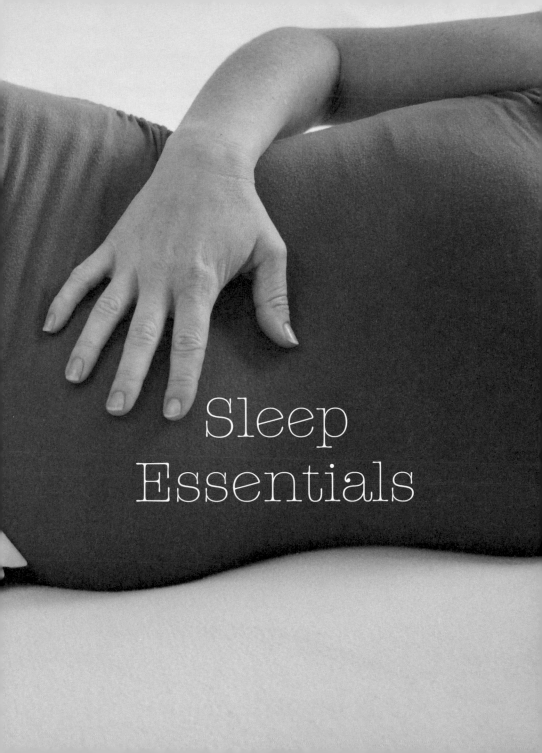

Sleep
Essentials

People who
say they sleep like
a baby usually
don't have one.

— LEO J. BURKE

WHY IS SLEEP IMPORTANT?

Sleep is an essential part of healthy living and is just as important as eating, drinking and breathing. When we have healthy sleep we feel, think and perform better. This is because sleep gives our bodies time to rest, restore, grow and strengthen. Sleep allows our bodies to maintain a strong immune system to fight off illness and avoid diseases. It allows our brains to create and store memories and complete tasks quickly and accurately. Having better sleep also improves creativity and assists in regulating appetite.

Importantly, sleep plays a big part in balancing our emotions. As you may already know and feel, your pregnant body is incredibly busy. Work, family, friends and community commitments can also be demanding. With so much happening at this time in your life, it's easy for your mind to feel overactive and unsettled. The Australian Sleep Health Foundation says that sleep is 'a built-in biological source of resilience and the ability to bounce back'. Healthy sleep is a precious tool to help manage the demands of a busy life, stabilising how you feel. That's why it's essential to prioritise sleep, now more than any other time in your life.

WHY DO WE SLEEP?

After years of research, scientists still have different ideas as to why humans sleep. Four theories are listed here. The reasons why we sleep are most likely a combination of all of these.

Preservation	This is an early sleep theory that suggests simply that animals will find a safe place to sleep, hidden out of the way of predators.
Conservation	Another early theory that proposes the body has a break while we're asleep to let the batteries recharge.
Restoration	A theory that sleep allows the body time to restore: muscle growth, tissue repair and immune function renewal all happen while we sleep, and toxins created by the brain while we're awake are removed during sleep.
Processing and learning	This is a more recent theory that suggests sleeping gives the brain a break from outside stimulation so it has a chance to review the day's activities and process the information. This helps consolidate memories, which allows us to better retain and retrieve information in the future.

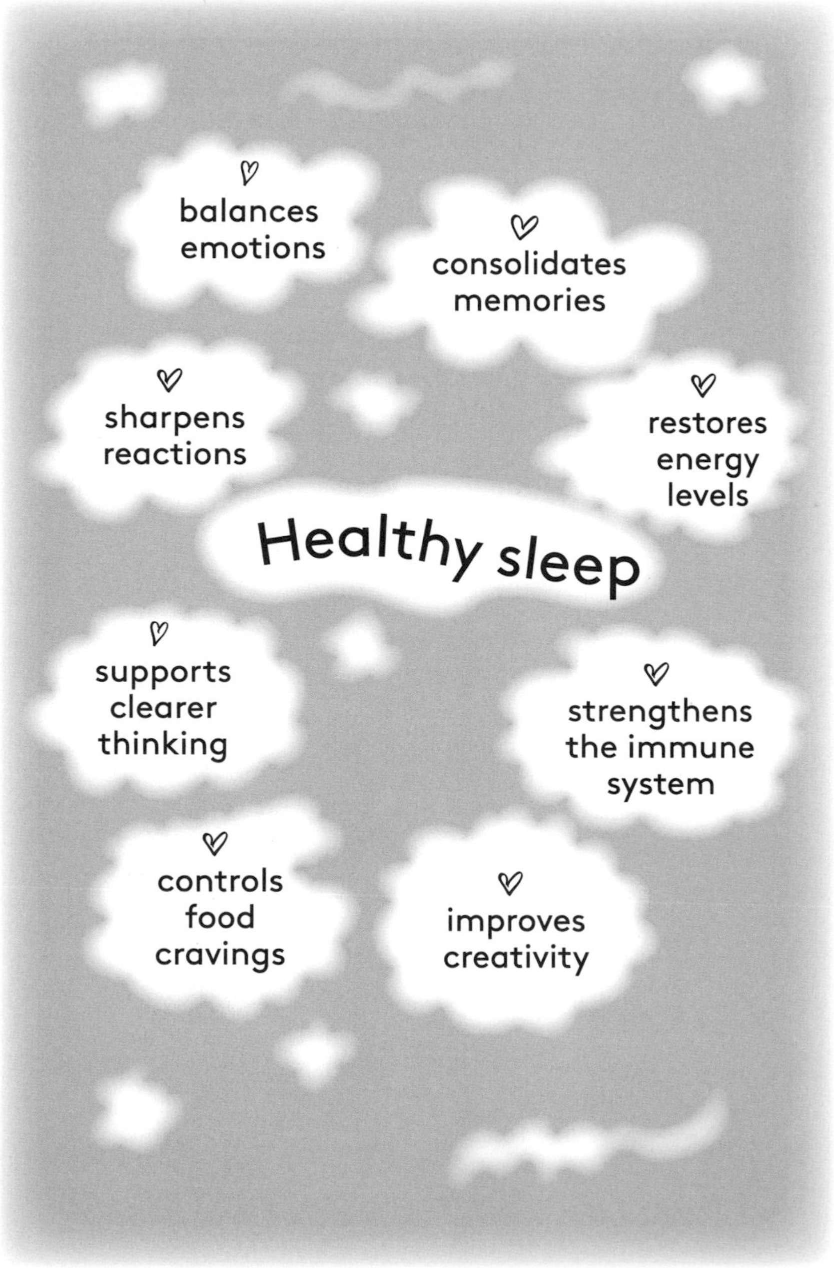

balances
emotions

consolidates
memories

sharpens
reactions

restores
energy
levels

Healthy sleep

supports
clearer
thinking

strengthens
the immune
system

controls
food
cravings

improves
creativity

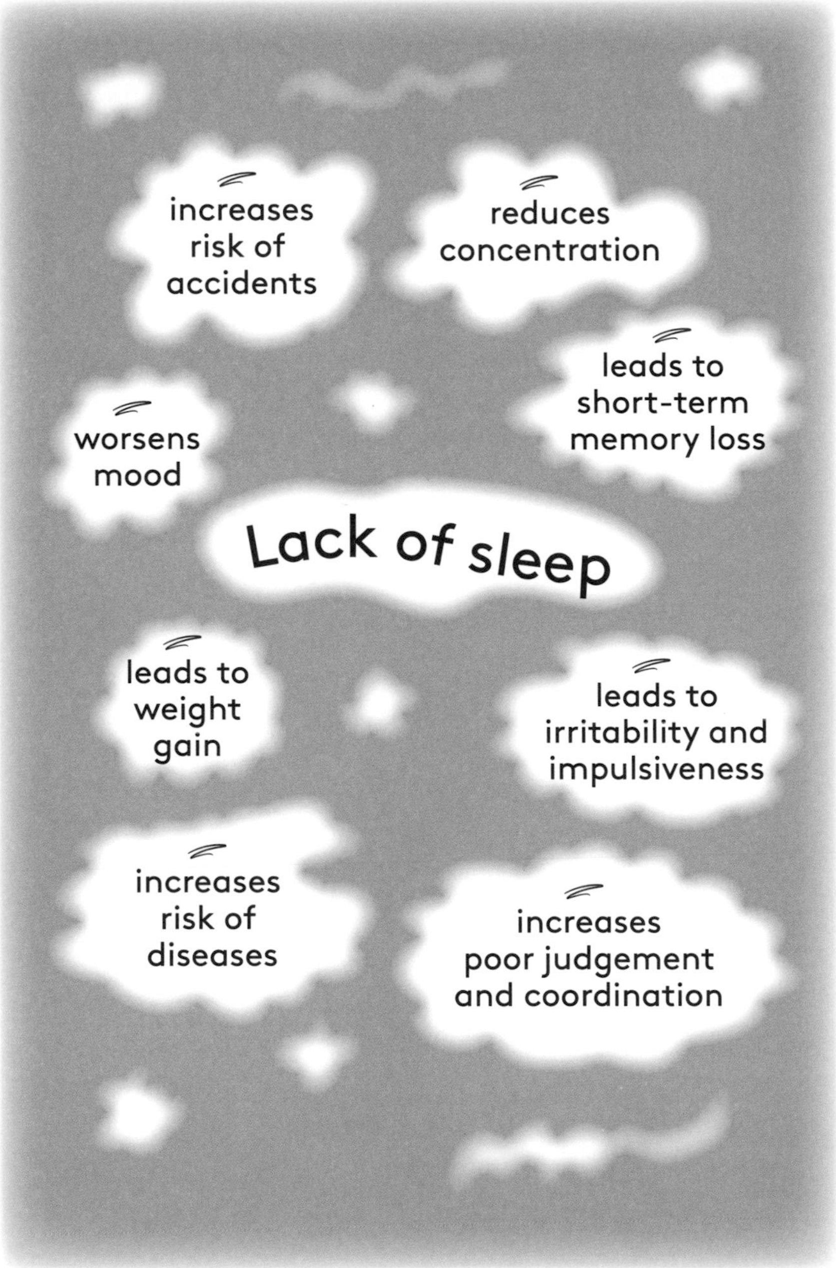
increases risk of accidents
reduces concentration
leads to short-term memory loss
worsens mood
Lack of sleep
leads to weight gain
leads to irritability and impulsiveness
increases risk of diseases
increases poor judgement and coordination

WHAT HAPPENS IF WE DON'T SLEEP WELL?

Poor sleep arises from getting too little sleep, disrupted sleep, sleeping at the wrong time, or a combination of all three. When our sleep is poor, we don't just miss out on the enormous benefits of healthy sleep; we can be affected by a range of negative consequences. It seems that some of these could affect your pregnancy, birth experience and your baby.

Acute sleep disruption/deprivation

If we don't get enough sleep, or we wake up a lot during the night, we experience sleep disruption. If we have just one or two nights of poor sleep, the sleep deprivation is acute (short-term) and we can experience a lack of focus, bad mood, sleepiness, headaches, or we can't remember or do things as well as usual. We can normally recover from acute sleep deprivation with a minimum of two good nights' sleep; however, it can take even longer to get back to performing at an optimal level.

> 24 hours of being constantly awake can result in the same level of impairment as a blood-alcohol concentration of 0.10%.
>
> (Williamson & Feyer, 2000)

Chronic sleep disruption/deprivation

When poor sleep extends into a few nights, sleep disruption becomes chronic (long-term) and the consequences can be more severe. As well as experiencing the symptoms above, long-term sleep disruption increases the risk of accidents, disease and disorders, and lowers our life expectancy. How sleepy we feel does not always reflect our actual level of sleep deprivation. Even though we think we are coping well, our health may still be affected.

How is sleep related to hunger, accidents and mental health?

Hunger	Are you hungrier when you're tired? Lack of sleep alters the release of hunger hormones, making the brain think we're hungry. Additionally, being tired means we might not have the energy to prepare and cook healthy meals; instead we might opt for a quick, high-calorie, processed option.
Accidents	Sleep deprivation decreases reaction time, concentration and the ability to make good decisions. This is because the area of the brain that is responsible for reasoning and judgement is vulnerable to poor sleep. This is especially relevant when we are doing activities where these skills are important, such as driving or doing complex work tasks.
Mental health	Sleep and depression share a bidirectional relationship: poor sleep increases the risk of poor mental health, and poor mental health increases the risk of having poor sleep. This is especially relevant if you have had mental health difficulties in the past. Improving sleep may help break this negative cycle.

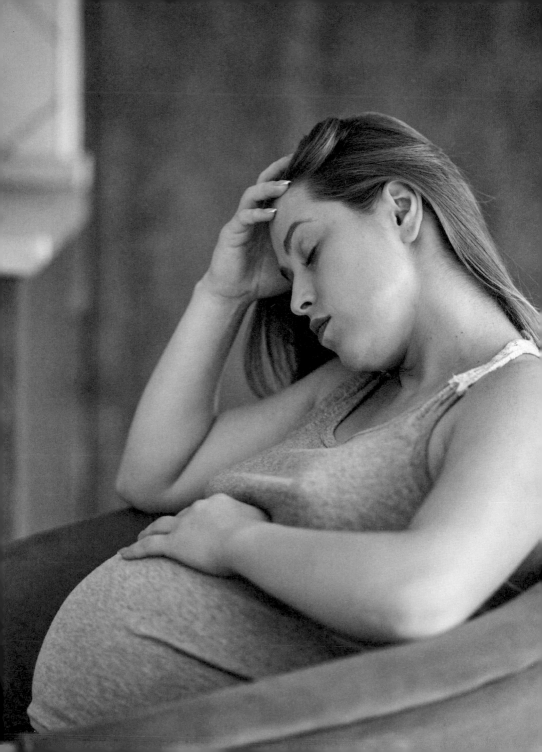

HOW DOES SLEEP WORK?

For centuries, it was thought our brains simply 'switched off' while we were asleep. But in the 1930s scientists were able to use an instrument called an electroencephalograph to measure electrical brain activity, and they discovered that humans' brain patterns change during sleep. More recently, researchers have discovered that sleep is highly regulated, complex and cyclical, and our brains are incredibly active when we sleep. Differences in brain activity help us categorise sleep into two types: NREM and REM.

When we sleep, we alternate between periods of NREM and REM about four to six times per night, with each cycle taking between 70 and 120 minutes. At the beginning of the night the cycles are generally shorter and we tend to have more NREM sleep and less REM sleep. As the night progresses, the cycles generally get longer and we have more REM and less NREM.

Sleep cycles

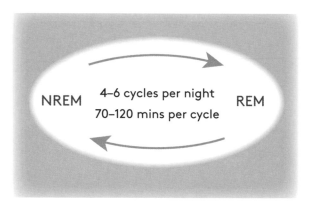

NREM ('non-REM') — Non-rapid eye movement sleep
REM — Rapid eye movement sleep

NREM and REM throughout the night

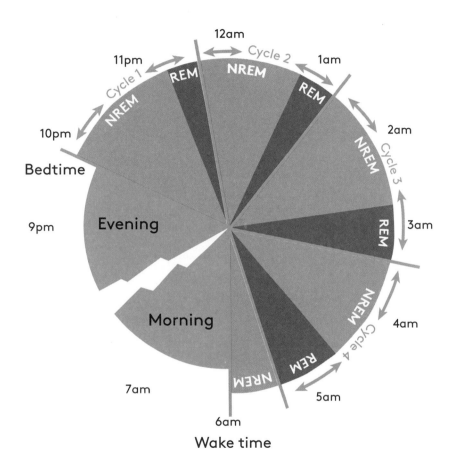

LIGHT SLEEP AND DEEP SLEEP

NREM sleep is further categorised into three types: NREM 1 (light sleep), NREM 2 (stable light sleep) and NREM 3 (deep sleep).

From light sleep through to deep sleep, brain activity becomes progressively slower.

If we look at just one cycle of NREM and REM from the last diagram, we can see how NREM is broken down into its different parts.

NREM 1, NREM 2, NREM 3 and REM are the four sleep stages we cycle through while sleeping. From being awake, almost everyone enters sleep through NREM 1, the transitional phase between wake and sleep. We spend only a short time in NREM 1, but it's long enough for our body to slow down and relax before moving into NREM 2. This is a more stable type of light sleep. It's here that the body temperature decreases and heart rate and breathing slow down. We then progress to NREM 3, the deep sleep stage. In this stage there are hardly any muscle movements and it's more difficult to wake someone.

REM sleep is a very active time for the brain and is the time when we have the majority of our dreams. This type of sleep is accompanied by periods of increased heart rate, increased blood pressure and, as the name suggests, rapid eye movements. However, while our eyes are moving, our bodies are almost completely paralysed — possibly a built-in protection mechanism so we don't act out our dreams! Body temperature is not well regulated during REM, which could explain why we can sometimes wake feeling hot and sweaty.

Sleep stages have different names: NREM 1 (N1 or Stage 1), NREM 2 (N2 or Stage 2) and NREM 3 (N3 or Stage 3).

Categories of NREM sleep

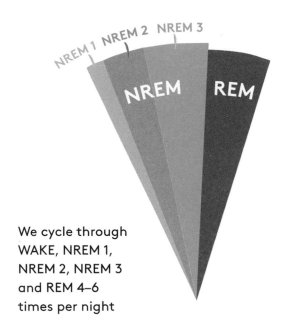

NREM 1   NREM 2   NREM 3

NREM   REM

We cycle through
WAKE, NREM 1,
NREM 2, NREM 3
and REM 4–6
times per night

NREM 1	NREM 2	NREM 3
light sleep	stable light sleep	deep sleep
N1 or Stage 1	N2 or Stage 2	N3 or Stage 3

Is one sleep stage more important than another?

Each sleep stage is just as important as another. It can be helpful to think about sleep as rooms in a house that you move in and out of. You would not get much done if you spent your whole day in just one room: you need to move into different rooms for different activities — for example, cooking in the kitchen, showering in the bathroom or watching TV in the lounge. Each stage of sleep has an important function, and cycling through each stage is how we get healthy sleep. The diagram below shows how we move through all the different stages during the night.

The stages of sleep throughout the night

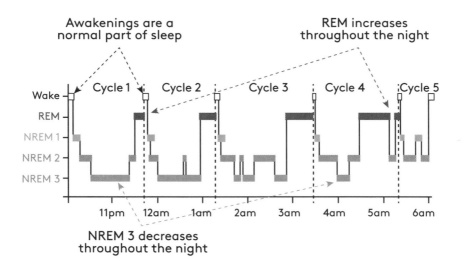

Adapted from Blume, del Giudice, Wislowska, Lechinger & Schabus, 2015

AWAKENINGS

You may have noticed the small periods of 'wake' in the previous diagram. Amazingly, while we're asleep, brain recordings show we can have up to 10–15 brief awakenings every hour. Most of the time, these awakenings only last a second or two and are so short we don't remember them. Sometimes, like in the diagram, they can last for a few minutes and we do notice them. It is completely normal to have up to three or four awakenings per night, even for healthy sleepers. Importantly, we can have these brief wake moments during the night without affecting our sleep health.

Sometimes, though, if the awakenings become too frequent, it can reduce the time we spend in NREM 3 or REM, which decreases our sleep quality. Alternatively, if the awakenings are too long, it can stop us getting the amount of sleep we need for good sleep health. This is important when you are pregnant, because the changes happening in your body can increase these awakenings. We'll see later on that there are some things we can do to help minimise sleep disruptions during the night.

WHY DO WE FEEL SLEEPY AT CERTAIN TIMES OF THE DAY?

Many processes on our planet occur with a regular pattern or rhythm; for example, the coming and going of the seasons, the ebb and flow of the tides, and the Earth's daily rotation, giving us day and night. Human sleep is guided by two regular body processes that work together to allow us to feel alert during the day and have a long, consolidated sleep at night. These two processes are the 'circadian clock' and 'homeostatic sleep drive'.

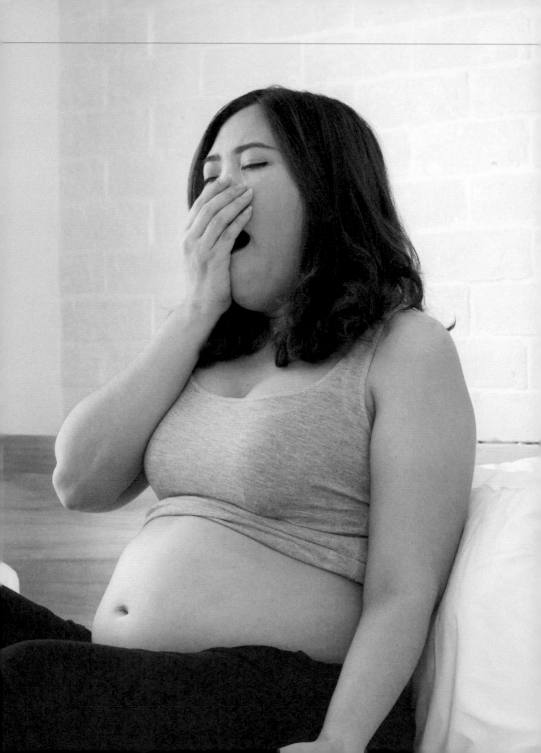

Circadian clock

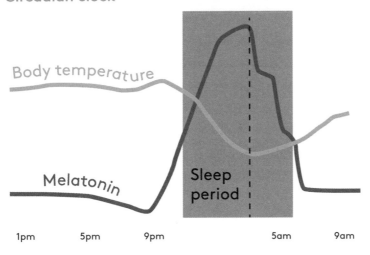

Body temperature

Melatonin

Sleep period

| 1pm | 5pm | 9pm | | 5am | 9am |

Adapted from Hickie, Naismith, Robillard & Hermens, 2013

Our body's circadian clock (sometimes called 'body clock' or 'circadian rhythm') regulates the timing of many systems in our body, such as eating patterns, body temperature, hormone production and — the most relevant for this book — sleep. The primary circadian clock is located deep within the brain in a region called the suprachiasmatic nucleus (SCN). This part of the brain gets information about light from special cells in the eyes. In the late evening, the circadian clock will reduce its wake signals and the body starts producing melatonin. When this happens, we start feeling sleepy. Melatonin levels in the body rapidly increase in the late evening, peak around 3–4am and rapidly drop again as morning approaches.

Body temperature is also closely related to sleep. A drop in body temperature happens at a similar time to falling asleep. Body temperature continues to drop during the night and is at its lowest when your melatonin levels are at their highest, again usually around 3–4am.

Wake maintenance zones

The diagram opposite shows how the wake and sleep signals from the circadian clock change over the day (the yellow line). These changes influence how sleepy we feel and also how awake we feel. Wake maintenance zones are:

* Blocks of time we are most awake
* Usually last 2–3 hours
* The first one occurs in the early evening (about 2–3 hours before bedtime)
* The second one occurs in the early to mid-morning (2–3 hours after waking)

Wake maintenance zones are when your circadian clock is sending out wake signals. This can make it difficult to fall asleep, or to stay asleep. On the other hand, your circadian clock has a mid-afternoon dip, when you are naturally sleepier: this nap window is when you are most likely to be able to fall asleep during the day. The exact timing of the wake maintenance zones can differ slightly from one person to another.

Homeostatic sleep drive

The homeostatic sleep drive is your body's urge to fall asleep after being awake for a certain period of time. The longer you are awake, the stronger the urge to fall asleep. The diagram on the next page explains this.

'Homeostasis' is our body's ability to keep itself balanced or stable despite what's going on around it. For example, body temperature: our body always tries to stay at around 37ºC, even though the external temperature might be much colder or hotter. Sleep is similar. The body wants to balance the amount of sleep and wake it has, so it creates a 'homeostatic sleep drive' to keep it balanced.

Wake and sleep signals

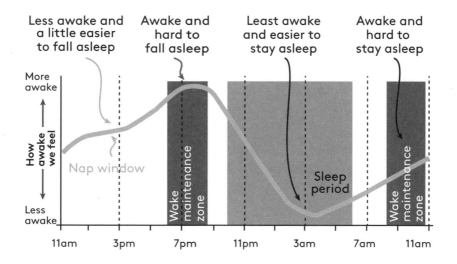

Adapted from Philippa Gander with permission

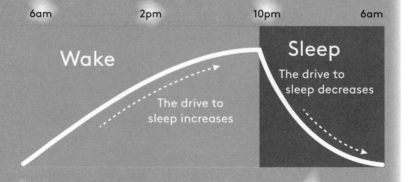

How do the circadian clock and homeostatic sleep drive work together?

The circadian clock and the homeostatic sleep drive work together to ensure you feel awake during the day and get a long period of sleep during the night. Late in the evening, both systems send strong signals to your body that it needs to sleep. Once you fall asleep, the sleep drive signal starts to decrease but the circadian clock sleep signal continues to increase. The circadian clock sends its strongest sleep signals around 3–4am. By around 6–7am your sleep drive is very low (because you've just had a long sleep!) and your circadian clock is sending stronger and stronger wake signals to your brain.

What type of circadian clock do you have?

The timing of our circadian clock is partly dependent on our genetic makeup. You may have heard people being described as 'owls' or 'larks'. 'Owls' prefer to go to bed later and get up later, while 'larks' like to go to bed earlier and wake up earlier.

Sometimes your circadian clock works well with your lifestyle and sometimes it doesn't. For example, if you don't feel sleepy until midnight but you need to wake at 6am to go to work, you may not be getting enough sleep. Or maybe you find it difficult to sleep past 5am, but your friends and family schedule activities that keep you up late at night. Again, you may find it difficult to get enough sleep.

WHAT AFFECTS OUR CIRCADIAN CLOCK?

Our circadian clock is mostly regular and predictable. However, many activities can influence it — some that we can control and others we can't.

Light

Light is the most important cue for our circadian clock: it helps it stay aligned with the day and night cycle of the sun. The effects of light on your circadian clock depend on when you are exposed to it — including to 'blue' light emitted from electronic devices such as computers, iPads, mobile phones, televisions, etc.

Being exposed to light in the evening delays the circadian clock cycle. This means that all the processes needed for falling asleep start later, including melatonin production. Delaying the circadian clock cycle also delays the waking up processes, so you will want to sleep later in the morning.

On the other hand, exposure to light in the morning advances the circadian clock cycle, making you want to go to sleep and wake up earlier. This advancing or delaying our circadian clock is called 'phase shifting'. Being able to phase shift our circadian clock cycle is sometimes beneficial because it means we can adapt to different time zones. But when we phase shift our clock with no change in time zone and we get too much light at the wrong time of day, it can cause serious problems for our sleep patterns.

Activities we can control

Bedtime routines

Eating & drinking

 Work & social activities

 Exercise

 Light 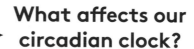 **What affects our circadian clock?**

Activities we can't control

Age

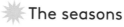 The seasons

Genetics

 Daylight saving

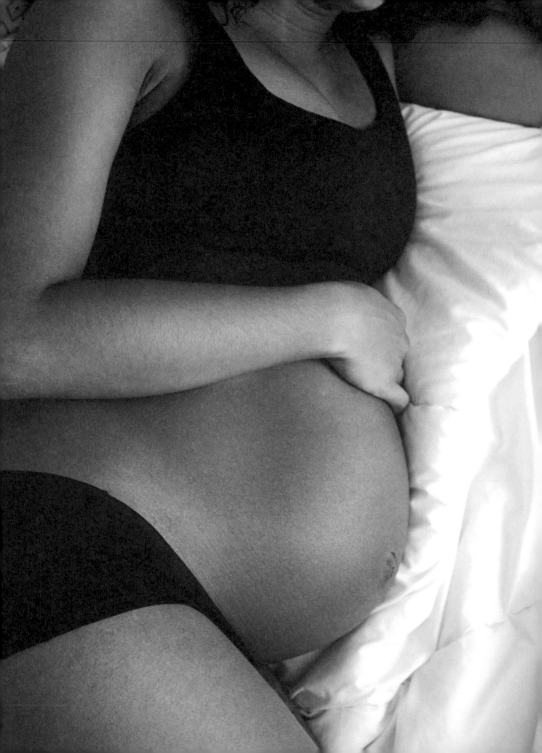

THREE STEPS TO GETTING HEALTHY SLEEP

There are three aspects of sleep that are really important for overall sleep health:

Sleep quantity	Is how much sleep you have in 24 hours. Healthy sleep quantity typically means getting 7–9 hours of sleep a night. Daytime naps can be included in the total amount.
Sleep quality	Relates to how refreshing your sleep is. It includes many different aspects of sleep such as quantity and timing, but also the time we spend in each sleep stage, how many awakenings we have and how long it takes to get to sleep. Your thoughts on how well you sleep are important when looking at sleep quality.
Sleep timing	Is when sleep is scheduled. It is influenced by whether you're an 'owl' or a 'lark'. Healthy sleep timing means keeping bedtimes and wake times as consistent as possible across the whole week — including weekends.

Sleep quantity

Most adults need 7–9 hours of healthy sleep per night to function at their best the next day. This varies among individuals: some need a bit less and others a bit more. Most of us have a sense of how much sleep we need, however it's very easy to function at a lower level during the day and think that it's normal — so it's important to re-evaluate how much sleep we need from time to time.

When we don't get enough sleep we do not need to make it up hour-for-hour. It takes a minimum of two full nights of good-quality sleep (going to sleep when you feel sleepy and waking up without an alarm clock) to return your sleep to normal. This can be difficult sometimes when you're experiencing sleep disturbances associated with pregnancy. If your 'sleep tank' is low, there are two strategies you can use to keep it topped up:

* Aim to spend longer in bed at night, as this is when your body is programmed for sleep.
* If night-time catch-up sleep is difficult, look for other sleep opportunities, such as daytime naps.

These two strategies might seem obvious, but we can all be guilty of putting sleep at the bottom of our priority list — often it just gets squeezed into our busy work, family and social schedules when time allows. But getting enough sleep is vitally important for both you and your baby.

Sleep quality

Sleep quality looks at how refreshing your sleep is — and it takes into consideration the whole sleep picture. Because it includes so many different aspects, people can have different views about what affects their sleep quality. For example, one person might find they are waking numerous times a night and believe this impacts their sleep enormously. Another person might also wake numerous times a night and it doesn't concern them, but the hour or two it takes them to get to sleep initially is a real problem for them.

Sleep timing

Remember that your circadian clock is influenced not only by light, but also by the patterns of your daily activities. Regular bed and wake times send important signals to your circadian clock, helping you to fall asleep when you want to and feel more alert when you wake up. When your body is prepared and expecting to sleep and wake up at consistent times, it transitions in and out of sleep more readily.

Consistent bedtimes and wake times means including your days off as well. Consider a workday week of Monday to Friday with weekends off:

Is this what your week looks like?

Monday, Tuesday, Wednesday and Thursday nights, you go to bed at 10pm and wake the next morning at 6am.

Friday night comes round and you think: 'Brilliant, I can sleep in tomorrow morning . . . I'll stay up tonight and finish my book.' So you stay up until midnight and sleep in until 8am on Saturday.

Saturday night rolls round and after a sleep in that morning, you don't feel so tired at 10pm. You think: 'I'll just watch one more episode of TV . . . I can sleep in tomorrow morning.' So you stay up until midnight and sleep in until 8am on Sunday.

Then on Sunday night you think: 'I have to get up at 6am for work tomorrow, I'd better get an early night . . .' But you don't feel so tired at 10pm and have trouble falling asleep. The alarm goes off at 6am on Monday and you don't feel so great . . .

A key to healthy sleep is consistency — making bedtimes and wake times as consistent as possible, even on weekends!

If your weekend bedtimes and wake times are one or more hours later than during your normal work week, you may experience 'social jet lag'. This change in bedtimes and wake times is telling your circadian clock to shift its timing, a bit like the 'phase shifting' we were discussing earlier. This is confusing for the body because it is effectively like changing time zones (hence the term 'jet lag') without a change in daylight hours.

Not only does social jet lag interfere with your sleep patterns (and makes waking up on Monday mornings difficult), but long-term misalignment between your sleep pattern and your circadian clock has been shown to increase your chances of developing heart, weight, digestion and mental health problems.

Timing

Do your bedtimes and wake times disrupt your sleep and daytime functioning?

Structure

Are you cycling through all the sleep stages and cycles?

Quantity

Are you getting 7–9 hours sleep per night?

Sleep satisfaction

Does your sleep allow you to function well during the day?

Daytime sleepiness

Do you find you are sleepy during the day?

Latency

How long does it take for you to fall asleep?

Awakenings

Do you wake too often during the night and does this affect how you feel during the day?

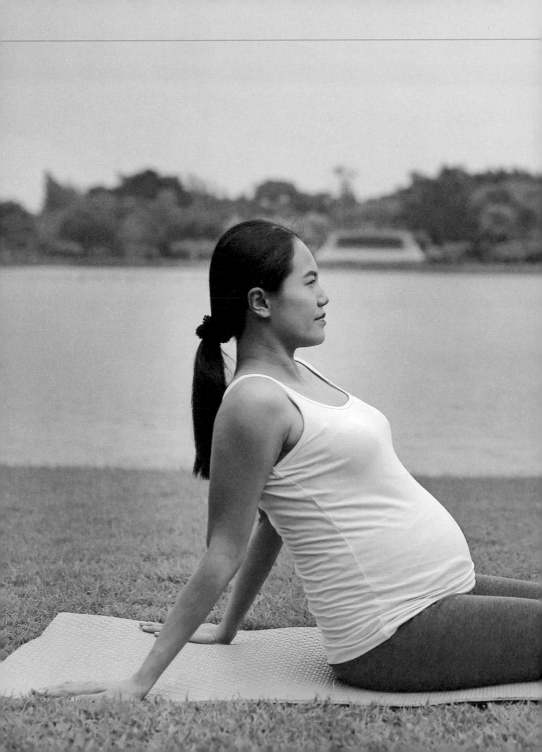

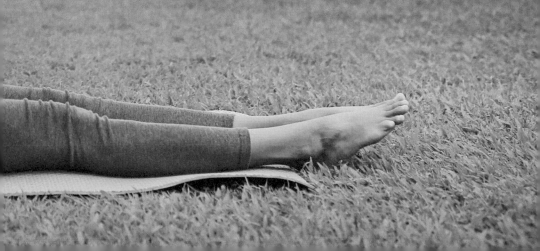
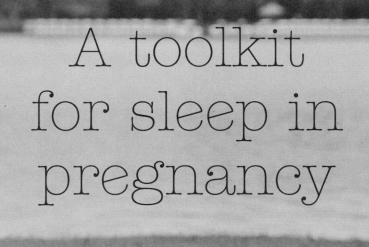

A toolkit
for sleep in
pregnancy

Without enough sleep, we all become tall two-year-olds.

— JOJO JENSEN

With all those changes happening in your body, it is completely normal to have changes in your sleep, too. In all likelihood, your sleep will be disrupted and it won't be quite the same as before you were pregnant. Having an understanding about what 'normal' sleep in pregnancy is helps to form realistic expectations about your sleep over the next few months. We can then work on getting the best sleep from the opportunities you have. We understand this can be challenging because you might be feeling tired, sore or nauseous, and being pregnant does not mean that work, family, household and social responsibilities can just be put on hold for an extended period of time. But it is an important time to pay special attention to your needs and prioritise your sleep.

Many factors can affect your ability to sleep while pregnant. Some sleep problems are short-lived and only slightly annoying. Other issues can continue for the duration of your pregnancy and are harder to manage. Each trimester brings new changes and challenges. In this section we'll look at some general strategies you can use throughout your whole pregnancy and then we will have a look at what's happening to your body in each trimester, and see why these trimester-specific changes affect your sleep.

Remember that the suggestions in this book form a toolkit of ideas and strategies you can choose from and experiment with.

Be open to trying some of these out. Healthy sleep can make a big difference to your pregnancy experience and can have substantial health benefits for you and your baby.

There are many sleep suggestions in this book. You may just like to try one at a time (if it is a big change) or try a few at the same time.

It can be helpful to reread these from time to time, including suggestions from other trimesters. Certain suggestions may fit better at different stages of your pregnancy or with how you're feeling at the time.

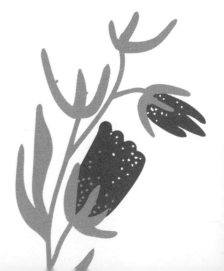

UNDERSTANDING AND SUPPORTING YOUR SLEEP

Your sleep may change	Be open and have realistic expectations about what normal sleep is in pregnancy.
Take some time to think about your sleep	What works well with your current sleep habits, rhythms and environment? What could be better?
Prize and prioritise sleep	Look for ways to maximise your sleep opportunities during the day and during the night.
Plan for sleep	Just as you might plan and schedule the rest of your life — it's a way of signalling to yourself and those around you that you take sleep seriously.
If things get tough	Please contact your healthcare provider — there are lots of people who can help you.

SLEEP MEDICATION

If you are experiencing a particularly bad patch of poor sleep, it may be tempting to take sleep medication. While occasional use of certain medications may be considered safe during pregnancy, some sleep medications have been linked to negative health outcomes for the baby. It is crucial that you speak to your healthcare provider before taking anything and be sure you are educated on the risks and side effects.

SLEEP DURATION AND SLEEP OPPORTUNITIES

In our busy lives, finding time for sleep is not always easy. But if you are constantly feeling tired, the first two questions to ask are:

* How much sleep do you need to function well during the day?
* How much time do you actually set aside for sleep?

It may seem like an obvious question, but are you giving yourself long enough for the amount of sleep you need? Are you going to bed at a reasonable time, or are you staying up late to fit more into your evening? If so, do you need to go to bed earlier? Are you getting up early to find extra time in the day? If so, do you need to sleep later?

Knowing how important sleep is while you're pregnant, now is the time to ensure your sleep opportunities are long enough to fulfil your sleep requirements.

Find time for a daytime nap

Napping can be very helpful to increase how much sleep you're getting, especially if your night-time sleep is not as good as it could be. A short nap can improve alertness for a few hours, which can be hugely beneficial to get you through the afternoon and evening.

Pregnancy is a really good time to start trying daytime naps. Once your baby arrives, your sleep will be disrupted for a few weeks (or years!) and napping is a valuable way to keep your sleep tank topped up. Given what we know about our circadian clock, having a nap can actually be tricky. You may not be used to napping, or maybe it's hard to fit into your work/family schedule — but give it a try. Even if you don't get the sleep you need, just having a rest can be valuable.

Daytime naps — here are a few tips:

If you nap regularly, try to nap at the same time each day. Sleep comes more easily if your body is expecting it.

We are naturally less alert in the mid to late afternoons. If this is a suitable time for a nap, you may find it is easier to nod off.

Try taking your nap in a dark place with a comfortable temperature. Close the curtains or wear an eye mask to make it as dark as possible.

Minimise the chance of interruptions to your sleep. Turn your mobile phone off or to silent, if possible, and maybe put a sign on the door to let people know you're resting.

Give yourself a 40–45 minute sleep window: this will hopefully allow a 30–35 minute nap. For some, sleeping for any longer can leave you feeling groggy when you wake. For others, if you find you have the ability to fall asleep, you may be able to sleep longer and still wake feeling refreshed. It is important that you don't sleep too late in the afternoon, as it may affect your ability to fall asleep in the evening.

If your daytime naps are affecting your night sleep, stop for a few days or weeks and see if your night sleep improves. You can always try a napping strategy later in your pregnancy.

SLEEP TIMING — CONSISTENT RHYTHMS

Remember, consistency is key! Going to bed and waking up in the morning at the same time every day makes it more likely that you'll get the amount of sleep you need. Consistent bedtimes and wake times reinforce the circadian clock's sleep/wake signals, allowing sleep to come more readily and helping you wake feeling more alert.

The following activities will help with consistent sleep

Set your bedtimes and wake times to the same time each day, even on weekends. It can be helpful to work backwards:

* Work out what time you would like your wake time to be, making sure you leave enough time for all your morning activities.
* Once you have a wake time, work backwards 7–9 hours (depending on how much sleep you need to function well during the day). This will give you your actual bedtime. Remember, though, you may struggle to fall asleep if your bedtime is in your evening wake maintenance zone.
* Start your bedtime ritual 30–60 minutes before your actual bedtime.

Try to get some exercise on a daily basis, such as walking or yoga.

If you are doing more vigorous forms of exercise, try doing it in the morning. Avoid doing any vigorous activities 2–3 hours before bedtime.

Practise a relaxing bedtime ritual that prepares your body and brain for sleep. So often in the evenings we rush around with jobs or chores or jump on to screens to check social media, emails or texts. Our bodies are still energised and our minds are still engaged, so it's not surprising that it's difficult to switch off.

* Create a routine. About 30–60 minutes before your planned bedtime, spend some time in quiet, non-stimulating activities such as reading, having a bath or shower, craft work or listening to music or a relaxation app.
* Think of these precious well-earned minutes as 'me time'.

Open your curtains or blinds wide when you wake up and keep them open during the day to let bright light in. Natural light exposure helps our circadian clock to line up with the day/night cycle.

Try to spend time outdoors in the sunlight every day.

Try not to fall asleep on the couch in the evenings — this reduces your sleep drive and can make it harder to fall asleep when you do go to bed.

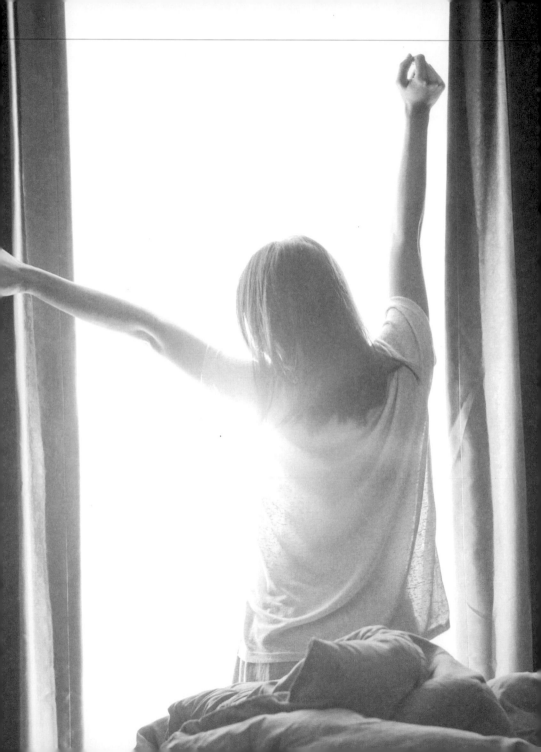

SLEEP QUALITY — MAKING YOUR BEDROOM SLEEP FRIENDLY

Light

Light (even artificial light) is a powerful cue for your body to be awake.

* Avoid bright light for 1–2 hours before bed. Televisions, computer screens, mobile devices and brightly lit rooms are sources of light, which can delay your circadian clock and the processes that are needed for falling asleep.
* Consider using low-wattage incandescent lights in areas you spend time in before sleep, such as the bedroom and lounge.
* At night, turn the lights off in your bedroom and check what light is sneaking into the room, such as from a streetlamp, porch light or sensor light, standby lights from electronics or alarm clocks. Try to block these light sources where possible.
* Avoid turning the bathroom light on when you get up at night, as this sends wake signals to your brain. A non-LED nightlight in the bathroom can be a good solution.
* In the summer months, use curtains or blinds to block out early sun so you can continue sleeping until your usual wake time. In the winter months, open the curtains after your normal wake time so the morning sun can provide a regular light cue to your circadian clock.
* If you are a shift worker, manage the light in your home to make it easier to sleep during the day. Ensure there is low light when you are winding down for sleep and limit the use of light-emitting screens. When you're trying to sleep, use blockout curtains or an eye mask to ensure that light signals are not being sent to your circadian clock.

Sounds

Sounds during the night can disturb your sleep. You may remember a loud noise that has woken you up, but even soft noises could be disturbing your sleep and impacting your sleep quality.

* Turn your mobile off or to silent, as the alerts may be enough to wake you. If you use your mobile for an alarm in the morning, switch it to silent first or put it in flight mode — or try a traditional alarm clock.
* If you're using an alarm, consider a sound that will wake you but not startle you. You want to start the day alert but not alarmed.
* If loud noises are causing you to wake, try finding a white noise that works for you (and your partner) and experiment with the volume. White noise works by reducing the difference between loud sounds (a truck passing, a partner's snoring or a dog barking) and background noise. Anything with a constant, soothing sound may work, such as a fan or a heat pump (TV and music have constant changes in tone and volume, so are not suitable). Try one of the white noise apps available to download.
* Earplugs can be useful to block any unwanted noise, but they may take some time to get used to.

Room design

Going to bed is a time for your body to have a break after a busy day. Making your bedroom feel comfortable and peaceful will help you feel relaxed and ready for sleep.

* Try to make your bed as inviting and cosy as possible.
* Is your mattress comfortable and supportive? Most good-quality mattresses will last around 9–10 years.

* Ensure the path to the bathroom is clear during the night so you don't have to turn lights on to see where you're going.
* When we use bed for sleep and sex only, the process of climbing into bed will naturally start the brain thinking it's time for sleep. Avoid working onscreen or watching television in bed. If you enjoy reading before bed, try sitting in a comfy chair rather than in bed.

Overheating

Generally, people get a better night's sleep in a cooler room, at around 16–19ºC. It's normal to sleep warmer when you're pregnant as your body is generating more heat from a faster metabolism, greater workload and higher levels of the hormone progesterone (which we will describe more in the next section).

Before you go to bed, think about the temperature in your bedroom:

* What season is it?
* What is the weather forecast?
* What bedclothes are on the bed?
* What are you wearing to bed?
* Does your partner's body heat affect you?
* Will you be running a heater during the night?

If you are waking during the night from overheating:

* Use a fan in the bedroom.
* Keep a window slightly open.
* Wear summer nightclothes.
* Swap the duvet for a lightweight blanket.

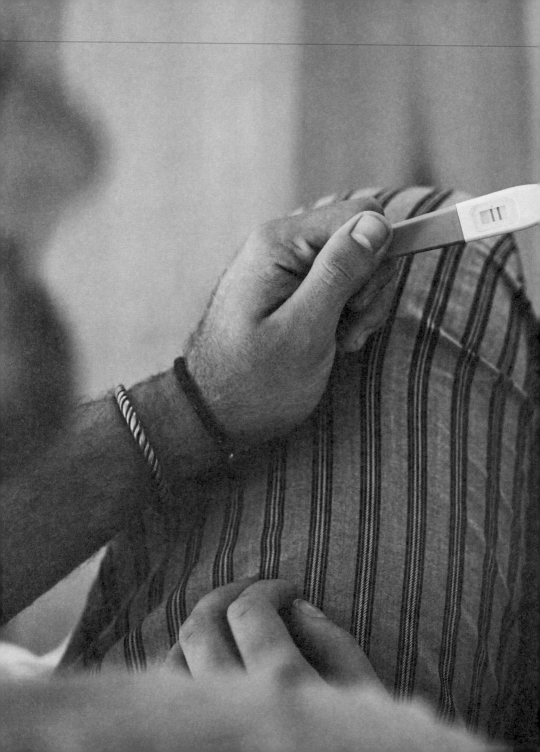

First
trimester

I used to get up
in the morning
feeling pretty good.
But now I'm pregnant
I can hardly get
through a day without
desperately wanting
to lie down for a nap.
I just feel so tired . . .

— VICKI (29)

Even though you may not look different on the outside, your body is undergoing some profound changes in these first three months. Your body is working hard, so it's not uncommon to feel significant levels of fatigue. This tiredness stems from two main causes: one is the enormous surge in hormones, which we'll look at next; and the second is greater disruption to your sleep from factors such as feeling nauseous, needing to go to the toilet often or having vivid dreams.

Tiredness can be tricky to manage, especially if you're not ready to tell people that you're pregnant, if you have busy work and family schedules, or you're feeling a bit worried or overwhelmed. But remember that sleep is closely linked to your mood, health and wellbeing, so protecting and prioritising your sleep right now is important. And it can result in some positive flow-on effects for you and your baby.

Remember that good sleep quality refers to sleep that has fewer disruptions, which helps you feel more refreshed on waking. During pregnancy, we know these disturbances are often hard to avoid, but the following suggestions may help you minimise the number and duration of sleep disruptions you experience.

HORMONES

Many hormones fluctuate in pregnancy. The main ones that affect sleep in the first trimester are progesterone, estrogen and human chorionic gonadotropin (hCG). These hormones are incredibly important for a healthy pregnancy, so it's vital to have them, but unfortunately they have some unwanted side effects on your sleep and energy levels.

Progesterone	
The upside	Progesterone production rises enormously at the beginning of pregnancy, as it is vital to keeping the placenta functioning properly and the uterus lining thick and healthy. It (in conjunction with another hormone called relaxin, see page 85) also plays a key role in keeping the muscles in the uterus relaxed so it can expand for your growing baby.
The downside	Progesterone makes you sleepy and increases your body temperature. It can also increase secretions from the sweat glands, making you feel hot and sweaty, which can disrupt sleep. Progesterone's role as a muscle relaxant is important for your expanding uterus, but it also relaxes other muscles and ligaments in your body, such as your digestion muscles. These usually contract to keep your food and gastric acids in your stomach. But when they relax, the contents of your stomach can move up into your throat and mouth, causing heartburn and reflux.

Estrogen	
The upside	Estrogen is the heavyweight of the pregnancy hormones: you'll produce more estrogen during one pregnancy than you will in the rest of your life. Estrogen increases blood flow in the placenta and uterus, which allows the transfer of nutrients to your baby and creates a healthy uterine lining. Estrogen stimulates your baby's hormone production, which triggers their organs to develop. Estrogen also promotes breast growth as your milk ducts develop.
The downside	The rapid rise of estrogen is thought to be the main reason why women can feel so nauseous in the first trimester (morning sickness). The severity and frequency of nausea varies enormously, and while it generally lessens in the second trimester, it can sometimes persist throughout pregnancy. Persistent nausea at any stage of your pregnancy can make you feel very tired. Your breasts feel tender as they grow, and this can make it difficult to find a comfortable sleeping position, or you may find you wake at night. Finally, estrogen can trigger mucous production, which can affect your sleep by causing nasal congestion when you're lying down.

Human chorionic gonadotropin (hCG)	
The upside	hCG is another hormone produced early on in pregnancy — and it is the ringleader! It tells your body you have a fertilised egg about to grow. hCG triggers the production of estrogen and progesterone in the ovaries, and it also tells the ovaries to stop producing eggs for the next several months. In the first 10 weeks hCG levels nearly double every 48–96 hours, and around the 10–12 week mark levels start to decline. hCG is the hormone that pregnancy tests detect to determine if you are pregnant or not.
The downside	Along with estrogen, it is thought that high hCG levels could be the reason why so many women suffer from morning sickness. As mentioned previously, nausea and vomiting can be hugely fatiguing and affect how much energy you have.

NAUSEA

Nausea is quite common in the first trimester and you may feel nauseous as soon as you wake up or sometimes, annoyingly, before you're ready to wake up. Although it's called 'morning sickness', nausea can occur throughout the day and during the night, which can be incredibly tiring. Feeling tired can often make the nausea worse, so it's important to prioritise your sleep and rest. There are lots of different ideas for how to minimise nausea: some work for some women and not for others. Keep trying until you find something that works for you. Suggestions include:

* Eat small amounts of nutritious foods often throughout the day.
* Eat foods that are high in carbohydrates or protein, like rice, potatoes or pulses (e.g. chickpeas, beans, lentils).
* Have a bland snack such as crackers or dry cereal next to your bed that you can eat as soon as you wake.
* Get out of bed slowly and let your body adjust to being upright.
* Avoid triggers that make you feel sick, such as certain smells or tastes.
* Drink small amounts of fluid or suck on ice chips throughout the day and in between meals, rather than with food. Try both cold and warm drinks to see what makes you feel better. It is especially important to keep your fluids up if you're vomiting.
* Ginger has been shown to reduce nausea and vomiting in pregnancy. Use ginger in your cooking, and drink ginger tea, ginger ale or ginger beer (non-alcoholic) or ginger syrup — all of these may help. But if you intend to take ginger supplements, please talk to your healthcare provider as there may be interactions with some medications or potential side effects with certain doses or products.

If nothing helps, talk to your healthcare provider as you may need further help for your nausea or vomiting. Prescription medications are available if symptoms are severe.

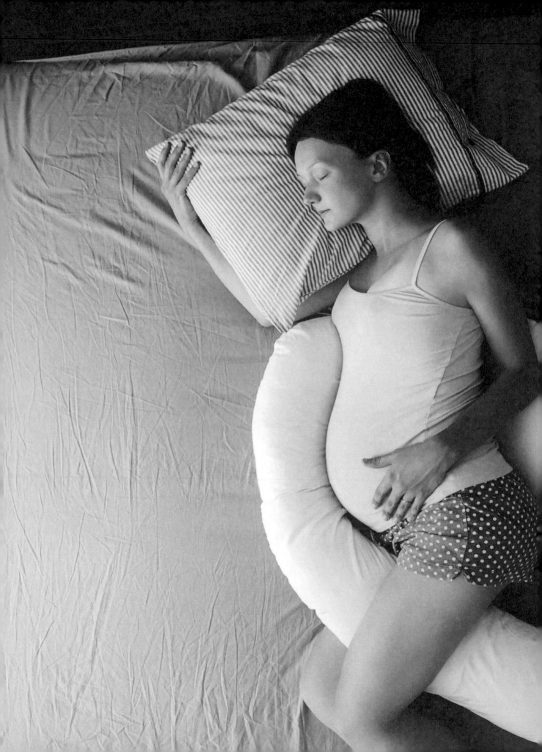

TOILET TRIPS

You may find you need to get up to go to the toilet during the night — maybe even several times.

* As mentioned previously, try not to turn the bathroom light on as this sends wake signals to your brain. A non-LED nightlight in the bathroom can light your path to the toilet safely, without overly waking you. Just make sure the way is clear of obstacles before you go to bed!
* It's extremely important to drink about 2–3 litres of fluids during the day as this helps your body absorb nutrients, transport blood and oxygen around the body, get rid of waste products and prevent constipation and dehydration. But try cutting back on fluids 2 hours before bedtime, and ensure you go to the toilet just before going to bed.

SLEEP POSITION

Although it's not as vital in the first trimester (as your baby isn't heavy yet), it's important to start trying to go to sleep on your side from 28 weeks gestation. This is especially relevant now if you are a back or tummy sleeper, as you may need time to adjust to a different sleep position.

A number of studies have shown that going to sleep on your side can lower the risk of stillbirth. This is because when you sleep on your back, the weight of your baby and uterus can restrict the flow of blood in the inferior vena cava — a large vein that takes blood from your feet back to your heart.

However, it's important to remember:

* We are talking about the position you go to sleep in, as this is the position in which you'll spend most of your sleeping time.
* Don't worry if you find yourself waking up on your back. Shifting positions is natural during sleep. Just settle on your side again to go back to sleep.
* Side sleeping is advised for any day or night sleeps.

There are a couple of ways to sleep more comfortably on your side. Try lying with your legs and knees bent, with a pillow between your knees and a pillow under your tummy. You could also put another pillow behind your back to provide more support, and to prevent you rolling onto your back while sleeping.

FOOD AND DRINK

We have seen how your sleep affects your metabolism, hunger and choice of food. The reverse is also true: what you eat and drink affects your sleep.

* Avoid caffeinated foods and drinks for a minimum of 5 hours before bedtime. This includes tea and coffee, chocolate, cola and energy drinks.
* Aim to eat your evening meal 2–3 hours before bedtime. If you find you are hungry later in the evening, have a small snack only.

BREAST PAIN

If your breasts are getting tender, try wearing a bra that is comfortable and has plenty of support. Your breasts are likely to increase in size during pregnancy, so you may need to check your bra size. Wearing a soft crop top bra to give some support may help with breast tenderness while you sleep.

BACK PAIN

Approximately one in every two women will experience some level of back pain in pregnancy. Symptoms can be common in all trimesters, primarily from hormones in the first trimester, and from your growing baby in the second and third trimester. The intensity of pain can interfere with many daily activities, and especially with sleep.

Some things that may help include:

* Aquarobics (gentle exercise in water).
* Pregnancy yoga or a Pilates class.
* Regular low-impact exercise such as walking.
* Avoid wearing high-heeled shoes.
* Use support pillows while sleeping.
* Maintain your posture and be particularly careful with lifting and twisting.

A heatpack on the painful area may also help, but it is important to talk to your healthcare provider beforehand as you want to be careful about raising your core body temperature. Remember that if you are thinking about starting the exercises above, see your healthcare provider first.

Back pain in pregnancy should not be ignored and it is important to talk to your healthcare provider as they may be able to refer you to a women's health physiotherapist for treatment.

PETS

Pets can be a source of sleep disruption, especially if they are sharing the bed with you, so consider their location at night. That said, many people find their pets a source of comfort, security and companionship. Research on this subject is mixed, so it's important to make the right decision for you.

INDIGESTION/HEARTBURN/REFLUX

Indigestion and heartburn can cause a burning feeling in your chest, and you may experience an acidic or bitter taste in your mouth (reflux). This is particularly common in pregnancy: between 25 and 50 per cent of women will experience these symptoms. If indigestion, heartburn or reflux are causing problems, try these suggestions:

* Eat smaller meals more frequently, and eat slowly.
* Avoid large meals just before bedtime.
* Avoid spicy and fatty foods.
* Reduce caffeinated foods and drinks.
* Sleep on your left-hand side to keep your stomach lower than your oesophagus.
* Prop your head on pillows to keep your head higher than your stomach while you sleep.

If none of these work, ask your healthcare provider for suggestions.

NASAL CONGESTION OR PREGNANCY RHINITIS

If you have nasal congestion but no other symptoms (such as fever, sneezing, runny nose or a sore throat), and the congestion has lasted for six weeks or more of your pregnancy, it may be pregnancy rhinitis. This can affect up to 30 per cent of pregnant women. It can often appear very early on in pregnancy (thought to be caused by changes in your body's hormone levels), or it can suddenly start at any time throughout pregnancy.

Nasal congestion may cause snoring and, even if the snoring doesn't wake you, it can still disrupt your sleep. Try these ways to improve your breathing:

* Elevate your head in bed by using more pillows.
* Use nasal saline rinses or sprays (a saltwater solution that flushes the nostrils).
* Physical exercise.

If nasal congestion is having a noticeable effect on your sleep, or your partner says you're snoring, it may be a good time to consult your healthcare provider to discuss options.

If your stuffy nose is accompanied by other symptoms, or you're feeling unwell, get it checked out by your healthcare provider.

NIGHTMARES

Nine months may seem like a long time, but compared to a lifetime, pregnancy is quite short. Your brain is processing a huge amount of physical and emotional change in this relatively short amount of time, so it's normal for your dreams to feel more urgent, vivid or intense. Often the dreams pregnant women have are about their pregnancy or baby. It is very normal to have increased recall (remembering the dream after you wake), as well as feelings of anxiety and stress related to these dreams.

Up to 70 per cent of women will experience frightening dreams or nightmares at some stage during their pregnancy. If nightmares or dreams are causing you distress, it might be helpful to talk to your healthcare provider.

SLEEP DIARY

If you find you are having problems sleeping but are not sure why, record any notes in a sleep diary. It may show up some patterns that you have not recognised before, and you can always talk to you healthcare provider about these.

JUST CAN'T SLEEP!

Your mind might be very active with thoughts on being pregnant, the birth or becoming a parent. Maybe you're thinking a lot about financial, work or family concerns. Hormones also change the way your brain thinks, to prepare you for nurturing and protecting your baby. It's normal to feel overwhelmed, anxious, irritable or confused when you're pregnant.

It's not surprising that these thoughts will affect your sleep, too. Sometimes it's hard to put these feelings aside, and despite your best intentions and efforts, sleep just won't come. Staring at the ceiling can be immensely frustrating and can make it even harder to sleep. If you find yourself in this situation, work through the following steps:

* Try calming your mind by using breathing or relaxation techniques.
* If you don't fall asleep after 20–30 minutes, get up, find a quiet, warm, low-light place in another room (such as a cosy chair in the lounge) and do something quiet, like reading, meditating or listening to music. This is very important, because you want your bedroom environment to invoke feelings of sleepiness and not frustration.
* When you start to feel sleepy again (yawning, longer or more frequent blinking, etc.), try going back to bed.

GENERAL TIREDNESS

* Put your feet up during the day if you can — for example, in your lunch hour at work.
* You may hear family and friends say, 'make the most of your free time while you can', but it's important to balance social events with the rest and sleep your body needs.
* You may hear family and friends say, 'get some sleep, while you can': this is good advice!
* Say yes to offers of help: help with cooking and cleaning will give you extra time to rest.
* If you have any extra money in your budget, cleaning services may be helpful.
* Relax your household standards for the time being, if this gives you a chance to rest. If having an organised home is important to you, ask family or friends to help with jobs you don't mind handing over.
* Shop strategically and stock up on groceries for a week or two at a time, or consider online grocery services. This may be a good opportunity to set this service up, so it is established when your baby arrives.
* Meal planning, preparing meals earlier in the day or picking up a healthy takeaway option occasionally will give you time to rest in the afternoons or evenings when you may be feeling more tired.
* Avoid alcohol and smoking: as well as affecting your baby's health, they can interfere with your sleep.

ESTABLISHING A SLEEP PLAN

Decide what you'd like to change about your sleep. Be specific.

If it's taking a long time to fall asleep, try a 45-minute bedtime routine before your actual bedtime: for example, start at 9.15pm so you're ready for sleep at 10pm.

Work out what you need to do. For example:
* Make sure you can start preparing for sleep well before bedtime — i.e., you've finished with work, chores and other commitments.
* Ensure that your space is quiet, has low light, is a comfortable temperature and free from other household distractions.
* Have the items you need ready before the routine starts, e.g. relaxation app, a book to read, a blanket or a fan, PJs, and a snack for when you wake in the morning.

Plan your time:
* Have a shower.
* Relax in a chair with a book for 15 minutes.
* Hop into bed and listen to a relaxation app for 15 minutes.

Choose a time when you have the energy to truly commit to your plan. Plans are less likely to work if you're half-hearted about them.

Discuss your plan with your partner or other household members. It is good for them to know what you are planning and why, so they can give moral support.

Pick a few consecutive days that are free of social commitments so you can stick to your plan as closely as possible.

It may be helpful to record your sleep changes and how you feel over this time.

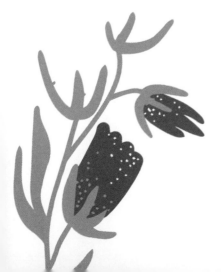

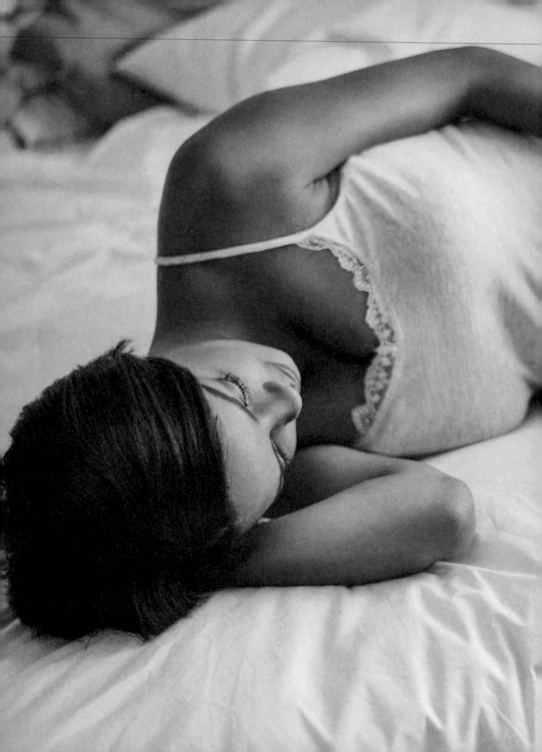

Second
trimester

Sleep is the golden
chain that ties
health and our
bodies together.

— THOMAS DEKKER

The second trimester may be welcome relief if you have had a difficult first few months. Your hormones are stabilising and for many women in pregnancy this means higher energy and less sleepiness compared to the first trimester. However, towards the end of the second trimester, some physiological events such as heartburn, nasal congestion, back, neck and joint pain, Braxton Hicks contractions, leg cramps or restless leg symptoms can start to disrupt sleep. Your baby's movements may start to wake you as they get bigger. The second trimester is also when many women experience vivid dreams — and snoring.

We are going to have a look at some of the strategies you can use to help you minimise these sleep disruptions. Remember there are some important strategies for sleep quantity and sleep timing in the toolkit section of this book that could help you get a good night's sleep, too.

SLEEP POSITION

If you can, keep trying to sleep on your side. This is going to become more important from 28 weeks gestation onwards, as the weight of your baby can restrict the flow of blood in the large vein (called the inferior vena cava) that takes blood back from the lower body to the heart.

For your main night sleep and any day naps, going to sleep on your side reduces the risk of stillbirth. But it's important not to worry if you wake up on your back: it's natural to change sleeping positions when you sleep. Just roll onto your side and go back to sleep.

Here are ways to sleep more comfortably on your side:

* Lie with your legs and knees bent, with a pillow between your knees and a pillow under your abdomen.
* Put another pillow behind your back to provide more support and to prevent you from rolling onto your back while sleeping.

LEG CRAMPS

Approximately 30 per cent of pregnant women experience leg cramps, especially in the second and third trimesters. Leg cramps are a painful contraction of the foot or calf muscle (or sometimes both). Even after the contraction subsides, the pain can linger for around 10 minutes.

If you are suffering a leg cramp, the best treatment for immediate relief is to flex the foot of the affected leg to release the contraction. Standing up and walking around can also be helpful, though you may need to hold on to something for balance initially.

For persistent leg cramps, it's unclear if oral supplements are effective. Some research shows that vitamin B, vitamin C, calcium or magnesium supplements can help reduce the frequency or severity of leg cramps, but other studies show no improvement. It's important to talk with your healthcare provider before taking these supplements.

> Quinine and vitamin E have been shown to have a positive effect on reducing leg cramps, but their use during pregnancy is not recommended.

Anecdotal evidence suggests that stretching, having a warm shower or applying hot or cold packs to the legs before bedtime can reduce leg cramps, but there is little research that shows this.

RESTLESS LEGS SYNDROME

Restless legs syndrome (RLS) (also known as Willis–Ekbom disease) is the irresistible urge to move your legs, usually to stop unpleasant sensations such as burning, itching or tingling. These sensations are often stronger when your legs are still, and especially when you are trying to sleep. About 10 per cent of the general population have RLS, but up to 30 per cent of women experience it during pregnancy, usually starting towards the end of the second trimester and through the third trimester. You're more likely to experience RLS if you're having your second (or more) baby, or if RLS runs in the family. Thankfully, most women find the symptoms of RLS disappear within days of their baby being born.

It is not yet known why RLS occurs, but hormonal changes, sleep loss and stress are thought to be contributors, as are low levels of iron and folate. If you think your iron levels may be low, or you have had low iron levels before you became pregnant, it would be helpful to see your healthcare provider.

Unfortunately there are no definitive guidelines for the treatment of RLS, but anecdotal evidence shows that massage, relaxation and stretching can help relieve symptoms. Because caffeine limits the absorption of folate, limiting caffeine intake can help, as will doing some exercise and avoiding alcohol. There are some medications that doctors can prescribe if your symptoms are severe, but be sure you know about the risks and side effects.

INDIGESTION/HEARTBURN/REFLUX

In the first trimester, indigestion is likely caused by increased levels of progesterone relaxing your muscles and slowing your digestion. But as you progress to the second and third trimesters your growing baby will increasingly push on the stomach and the oesophageal sphincter (the ring of muscle between your stomach and throat): together, the relaxed muscles and the increased pressure can force food and stomach acids into your throat, causing that burning sensation. This can become worse when you're lying down, because you lose the help of gravity to keep the food and acids in your stomach.

If you are experiencing problems with heartburn or indigestion, these suggestions may help:

* Eat smaller meals more frequently, and eat slowly.
* Avoid large meals just before bedtime.
* Limit spicy and fatty foods.
* Reduce caffeinated foods and drinks, including tea and coffee, chocolate, cola and energy drinks.
* Sleep on your left side so your stomach is lower than your oesophagus.
* Elevate your head with pillows, or use foam wedges or rolled-up towels underneath the head end of the mattress. This can take some of the pressure off the oesophageal sphincter during sleep and so limit the reflux.

BACK PAIN

Back pain can be common throughout pregnancy, but because your baby is getting bigger now, there are more muscular changes and fatigue, as well as shifts in your centre of gravity. The intensity of pain can interfere with many daily activities, and especially with sleep. Some things that may help include:

* Aquarobics or hydrotherapy.
* Pregnancy yoga or Pilates.
* Regular low-impact exercise such as walking.
* Avoid wearing high-heeled shoes.
* Use pillows to support your body while sleeping.
* Take care when lifting and twisting — you may not be able to lift or carry what you normally could.

Heat packs on the painful area may help, but talk to your healthcare provider beforehand as you want to be careful about raising your core body temperature. Remember that if you are just starting the exercises above, see your healthcare provider first. Back pain in pregnancy should not be ignored and it is important to talk to your healthcare provider as they may be able to refer you to a women's health physiotherapist for treatment.

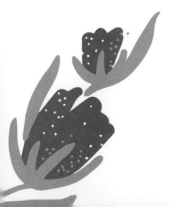

INSOMNIA

Insomnia is having difficulty with sleep, caused by problems falling asleep, staying asleep, waking up too early and/or not feeling refreshed after waking. Nearly half of all pregnant women worry about their sleep in the first and second trimester, or have some degree of insomnia during their pregnancy. This can increase to three-quarters of women in the third trimester.

It is very common to have a busy mind when you hop into bed. Maybe you're having anxious thoughts about the health of your baby, the labour and/or delivery, your work, or how you might balance work or finances with a new baby. Or you may be feeling excited about meeting your baby, getting baby clothes or thinking of names. Or you might just be thinking about remembering to book your next midwife appointment, wondering if that yoga centre has a pregnancy class, or maybe what to cook for your friends when they come for dinner tomorrow night.

An effective way to calm those busy thoughts is through the use of relaxation strategies, maintaining gentle but regular exercise routines, and reviewing the information we have discussed about your sleep patterns and behaviours, especially on bedtime routines. The Australian Sleep Health Foundation website has information that you may find helpful — see www.sleephealthfoundation.org.au/insomnia. Insomnia can be a complex problem, so it's an important time to talk to your healthcare provider if any of your worries or thoughts are causing you any concern.

Examples of mindfulness and relaxation apps		
Omvana	Smiling Mind	Mind the Bump
Insight Timer	Headspace	Calm

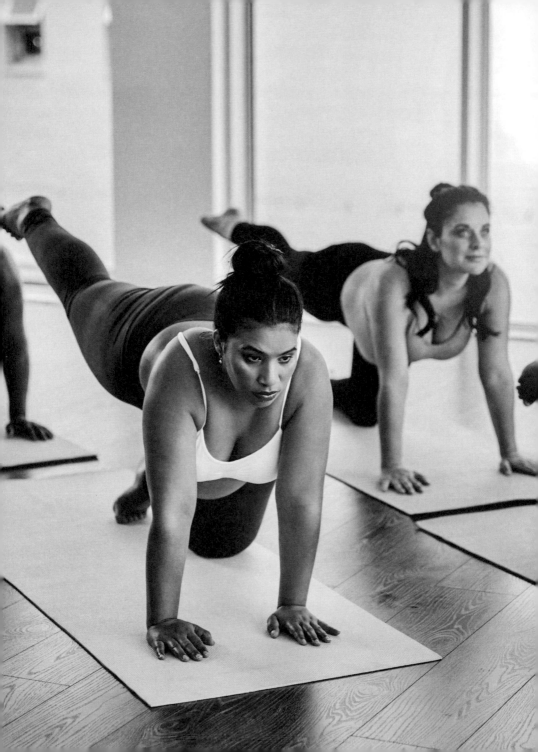

HORMONES

As you move into the second trimester, your hormones continue to fluctuate. Two of the most significant hormones at this time are cortisol and relaxin. As with all hormone changes during pregnancy, they play a vital role, but can also have downsides.

Cortisol	
The upside	Cortisol levels significantly increase later in the second trimester, and by the end of pregnancy levels are about two to three times higher than pre-pregnancy. Cortisol helps regulate the blood flow between the placenta and your baby, helps your baby's organs and brain to develop, and appears to have an effect on the start of labour. Cortisol is essential for you as the mother, too: it supports your metabolic system and helps your body manage stress and fight infections.
The downside	Cortisol production follows a circadian rhythm: typically it is at its highest levels when you wake up in the morning and lowest in the early evening. Elevated levels of cortisol over a long period of time, such as when you are experiencing extended periods of stress or poor sleep, can have an effect on your immune, metabolic and cognitive systems and can impact your baby's growth and development.

Relaxin	
The upside	Relaxin levels rapidly increase in the first trimester and reach a steady state in the second trimester. In early pregnancy, relaxin promotes foetal implantation and helps with the growth of the placenta and the lining of the uterus. It also helps with the increased demand for oxygen and blood flow, which further assists nutrient and waste removal in the heart, kidneys and placenta. Later in pregnancy, relaxin assists with the softening of the cervix and relaxing of the ligaments around the pelvis, to help the childbirth process.
The downside	The role of relaxin as a muscle and blood vessel relaxant may soften the upper airway muscles during sleep. If this restricts the flow of air from your nose and/or mouth to your lungs it can increase the chance of snoring or breathing problems, especially later in pregnancy. The relaxant properties of relaxin on the back muscles and ligaments are thought to be one reason why women experience increased back pain during pregnancy, as there may be greater instability or misalignment in joints or a shifting in posture.

BREATHING

The increase in hormones, blood volume, oxygen demand and your growing baby throughout pregnancy significantly change the way your respiratory system works. The change to your breathing can be tiring, and it can cause breathing problems while you sleep.

Breathlessness

The increase in progesterone and estrogen changes the efficiency of your lungs and the amount of air you breathe in and out, which can leave you feeling tired. Your baby's growth also starts to restrict your diaphragm (the muscles between your chest and belly), and your lungs become squashed. This means it can be harder to get as much air in and out of your lungs — similar to feeling short of breath after exercising.

* It can be helpful to sit or stand up tall, and stretch your hands up towards the ceiling.
* Try a relaxation app or yoga that concentrates on breathing techniques.

If you are an asthmatic or have any type of respiratory illness during your pregnancy and you are worried it's affecting your breathing, please get in touch with your healthcare provider.

Nasal congestion

As mentioned in the previous section, nasal congestion (or pregnancy rhinitis) is fairly common in pregnancy. It may cause snoring and even if the snoring doesn't wake you, it still disrupts your sleep. Ways to improve your breathing might include:

* Elevating your head in bed by using extra pillows.
* Nasal saline rinses or sprays.
* Physical exercise.

If nasal congestion is accompanied by fever, sneezing, a sore throat or coughing, or if it's affecting your sleep, it's a good time to consult your healthcare provider.

Snoring and sleep apnoea

During pregnancy, many women snore more than normal. This is sometimes due to increased mucous production and also because your upper airway narrows and softens. If you or your partner have noticed heavy snoring, pauses in breathing or waking with a gasp, these could be symptoms of a sleep disorder called sleep apnoea. If this happens, it is important to speak to your healthcare provider. Sleep apnoea in pregnancy can increase the risk of having high blood pressure, diabetes and pre-eclampsia, which can affect your health and the health of your baby. Sometimes a sleep study may need to be done to see what is happening to your breathing while asleep.

Other strategies for dealing with sleep and fatigue

Put your feet up during the day if you can — it may help you have a bit more energy later in the day.

Try to balance social events with the rest and sleep your body needs.

Say yes to offers of help with chores, cooking and cleaning — this will give you extra time to rest.

If you're not sure what is disrupting your sleep, try writing down your thoughts in a sleep diary. Note what you're eating, what times you are waking, thoughts you have when waking, etc. You may notice some patterns you haven't recognised before.

Your breasts may feel tender or be increasing in size. Check your bra is the correct size, and try wearing a bra that is comfortable and has plenty of support, such as a soft crop top bra, to help with breast tenderness while you sleep.

Is your favourite TV show on at 10pm? If you can, record it and watch it the next day or at the weekend. Thinking of watching that next episode in the series but know you should be going to bed? Try to resist — and get the sleep you need!

Consider the temperature in your bedroom at night. A cooler environment is more conducive to a good night's sleep.

Keep your weekday and weekend bedtimes and wake times as regular as possible — this reinforces your body clock's sleep/wake signals. Consistency throughout the week allows sleep to come more readily when the light is turned off and helps you wake feeling more alert in the morning.

Light and noise can disrupt your sleep, especially if you are moving through a light sleep stage, so make your bedroom as dark and quiet as possible.

If you can't get to sleep within 20–30 minutes, get up and go to another room. Find a warm, low-light place in another room and enjoy doing something quiet. When you start to feel sleepy again (yawning, heavy eyelids or itchy eyes), try going back to bed.

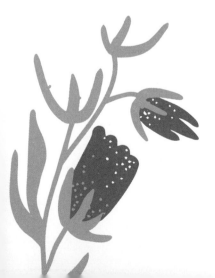

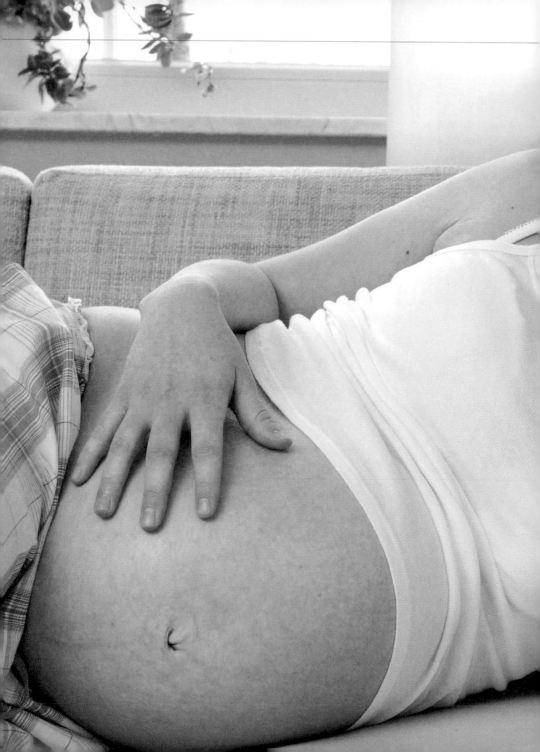

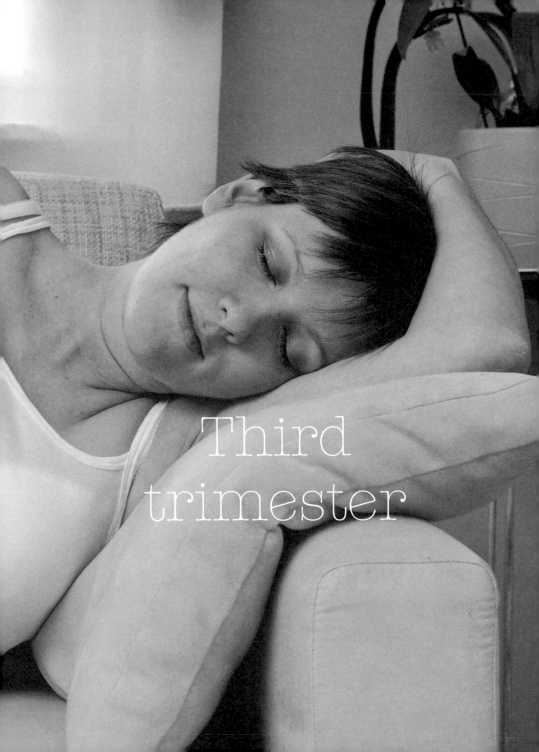

Third
trimester

Each month has between 28 and 31 days . . . except the last month of pregnancy, which has 1453 days.

— ANONYMOUS

You're on the home straight! While it can seem like your due date is approaching a little too fast, the last few weeks can also feel like they are never going to end. Getting good-quality sleep in the final trimester can be challenging. Your body is going through huge changes. Physiologically, it has to make room for your baby's rapid growth, and you will expend a huge amount of energy to keep up with your body's physical requirements. Emotionally, the countdown to labour and becoming a new mum can feel quite exciting but sometimes overwhelming, too.

Because of all the changes, your sleep can become more restless. Sleep is usually lighter in this trimester (with more time spent in NREM 1 and NREM 2 sleep and less time in NREM 3 and REM sleep), so it is easier to be awakened by noises that you would normally sleep through. In the third trimester, almost all women wake up multiple times — three times per night on average — and the awakenings usually last longer. This can leave you exhausted and drowsy during the day, and also affect your memory, concentration and mood.

Remember there are some important sleep quantity and sleep timing strategies in the toolkit section of this book that could help you get a good night's sleep.

HORMONES

As your body begins to prepare for the birth of your baby, hormones such as prolactin and oxytocin start to increase significantly.

Prolactin and growth hormone	
The upside	Prolactin is involved in breast growth, production of breast milk and strengthening the immune system. Towards the end of pregnancy, prolactin levels are 10–20 times higher than pre-pregnancy. Growth hormone is necessary for tissue repair, growth and metabolism in both the mother and baby. It is also at its highest levels at the end of pregnancy. Higher levels of both prolactin and growth hormone occur at night and play a role in enhancing and maintaining deep sleep.
The downside	None that we know of!

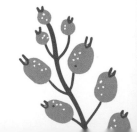

Oxytocin	
The upside	Oxytocin levels increase over the term of your pregnancy, and it is released in large amounts during labour. These high levels of oxytocin strengthen the contractions that open the cervix. After birth, oxytocin continues to stimulate contractions to promote blood clotting around the placenta. The oxytocin hormone is also released when your baby breastfeeds, encouraging the 'let down' of milk into the nipples.
The downside	In the last weeks of pregnancy, oxytocin is released in a rhythmic way, with lower levels during the day and higher levels at night. Oxytocin and melatonin (which is also present in higher levels during the night) act together to assist in the birth process. Higher levels of contractions also occur at night, and this is thought to be one reason why labour and delivery tend to occur during the evening hours. Sleep quality decreases progressively over the last five days of pregnancy and is lowest on the night before contractions and delivery start. Contractions during labour usually mean there is an extended period when you will be unable to sleep.

A WORKOUT FOR YOUR BODY

During the third trimester, your baby will be rapidly increasing in size. For women who are a healthy weight, this means you are carrying around 11–16 extra kilograms from your baby's weight, fluid, nutrients, breast and womb growth, placenta and blood volume. It's as if you're carrying an extra 6–8 two-litre bottles of milk around with you all the time. It's a big load for your body to move around all day. In fact, your body has increased its blood volume by approximately 50 per cent to deal with all this new growth. This means your heart is working hard to move that blood around. It's no wonder you're feeling tired!

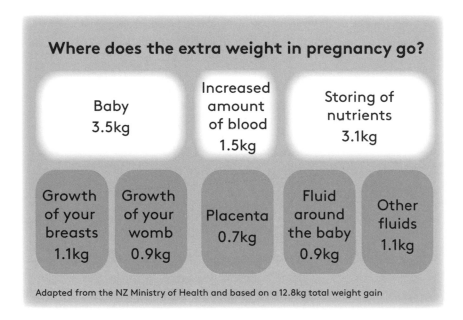

Where does the extra weight in pregnancy go?

Baby
3.5kg

Increased amount of blood
1.5kg

Storing of nutrients
3.1kg

Growth of your breasts
1.1kg

Growth of your womb
0.9kg

Placenta
0.7kg

Fluid around the baby
0.9kg

Other fluids
1.1kg

Adapted from the NZ Ministry of Health and based on a 12.8kg total weight gain

GENERAL TIREDNESS

Many women are maintaining a normal work and social schedule even while they're challenged with this increased physical load. In our busy lives, finding time for sleep is not always easy, but sleep and rest are vital for you at the moment. It can be helpful to revisit the questions we asked earlier:

* How much sleep do you need to function well during the day? This may be different to what it was pre-pregnancy or in the earlier trimesters.
* How much time do you actually set aside for sleep?
* Is your sleep opportunity long enough for the amount of sleep you need?
* Can you adjust your schedule to allow more time for sleep at night and/or rest during the day?
* It may be hard to ask for help, but you may be surprised at the positive response you get. Say yes if people offer to help: extra help gives you extra time to rest.
* It may not be easy to organise or accept, but can your life be a bit less busy for a while?
* Try to do work or household chores earlier in the day — this allows you to rest in the afternoons and evenings when you may be feeling more tired.

Find time for a daytime nap

If you have a few weeks between finishing work and baby's due date, this can be a great time to start trying to take consistent daytime naps. Taking a nap can increase how much sleep you're getting, especially if your night-time sleep is not as good as it could be. A short nap can improve alertness for a few hours, which can be hugely beneficial to get you through the afternoon and evening. Taking a nap is a valuable way to top up your sleep tank after your baby arrives.

Here are the napping tips from earlier in the book:

* If you nap regularly, try to nap at the same time each day. Sleep comes more easily if your body is expecting it. Consistency is key!
* During mid to late afternoon, we have a natural decrease in alertness. If this is a suitable time for a nap, you may find it is easier to nod off.
* Try taking your nap in a dark place at a comfortable temperature. Close the curtains or wear an eye mask to make it as dark as possible.
* Try to make sure your sleep is as uninterrupted as possible. Turn off your mobile phone if you can, and maybe put a sign on the door to let people know you're resting.
* Give yourself a 40–45-minute sleep window; this will hopefully allow a 30–35-minute nap. For some, sleeping for any longer than this can leave you feeling groggy when you wake. Others can sleep longer and still wake feeling refreshed. If you are finding it difficult to fall asleep at night, try cutting back on your nap duration or not napping every day.

It is important that you don't sleep too late in the afternoon, as it may affect your ability to fall asleep in the evening.

SLEEP POSITION

As we mentioned earlier, sleeping on either side helps lower the risk of stillbirth and assists the flow of blood and nutrients to your baby and uterus. However, it's important not to worry if you find yourself waking up on your back. Shifting positions is natural during sleep, and it is the 'going to sleep' position is most important. Just settle on your side to start your sleep again. Side sleeping is advised for any sleeps, including naps.

Most women find they are most comfortable on their side with pillows for support. Experiment with pillows between your knees, under your abdomen or behind your back to discover a comfortable position.

WHY AM I GOING TO THE TOILET SO OFTEN?

Extra work for your kidneys	The increased blood and fluid moving through your body means your kidneys are filtering more too. Increased filtering increases the amount of urine being produced. More urine means more toilet trips.
Relaxed muscles in urinary system	Progesterone and relaxin are hormones that relax muscles and ligaments to help cater for your expanding abdomen. However, these hormones also relax the muscles around your bladder, making toilet trips more frequent.
Increased pressure on your bladder	As your baby grows, the pressure on your bladder increases. This can make it seem like you need to urinate even if your bladder is empty. This feeling intensifies as you baby's head becomes engaged ready for birth.

Here are some things that may help:

* The pressure on your bladder causes it to change shape. This can make it difficult to fully empty when you go to the toilet and make you feel like you need to urinate soon after. Try leaning forward or rocking back and forth while urinating to help your bladder empty.
* Don't reduce your fluid intake, even though the constant trips to the bathroom can be annoying. It's crucial for you and your baby's health to stay hydrated.
* Cut back on caffeinated drinks as these increase the production of urine.
* To reduce the number of toilet trips during the night, drink plenty of fluids in the morning and afternoon, but start to reduce fluid intake two hours before bedtime and go to the toilet just before going to bed.

BABY'S MOVEMENTS

Ironically, your baby may be particularly active at bedtime, just as you are settling in to sleep. This may be due to your body movements during the day gently rocking the baby to sleep, or maybe you're more aware of baby's movements when you're still. Either way, your baby's 10pm disco party can be distracting when you're trying to sleep.

If the movements are stopping you from getting to sleep, you could try moving to another position for a short time to see if your baby settles.

Anecdotally, women have found that their baby's movements increase after eating and drinking, though there is limited research on this. You could try avoiding food and drink just before bedtime.

BRAXTON HICKS CONTRACTIONS

Braxton Hicks contractions are false labour contractions. It's your body's way of rehearsing for labour and childbirth. The contractions are a tightening of the uterus muscles, which makes your belly feel hard. They are normally irregular and usually painless, though they can be quite uncomfortable as the muscles tighten around your abdomen. Some women never feel Braxton Hicks contractions and others experience them for weeks before labour starts. These contractions certainly have the ability to disrupt your sleep if they occur throughout the night.

* Try moving to another position for a short time to see if the contractions lessen or stop.
* Dehydration can trigger Braxton Hicks contractions, so ensure you are getting plenty of fluids during the day.

SNORING

As we have discussed previously, snoring is common in pregnancy, and some studies show that the frequency of snoring doubles in the third trimester compared to pre-pregnancy levels. This can be due to increased mucous production and also a softening and narrowing of the upper airways, which can restrict the flow of air in and out of your lungs.

If your partner mentions that you're snoring heavily, or that you have times when your breathing pauses, or you have woken up from sleep with a gasp, then it's important to speak to your healthcare provider so they can assess you for a sleep disorder called sleep apnoea. Sleep apnoea in pregnancy can increase the risk of having high blood pressure, diabetes and pre-eclampsia, which can affect your health and the health of your baby. Sometimes a sleep study may need to be done to see what is happening to your breathing while asleep.

BACK PAIN

Several things can cause back pain in the third trimester, including softening of the ligaments and muscles (which can lead to joint instability), carrying around 11–16 extra kilograms in weight, and changes in your centre of gravity. These changes can make you feel less steady on your feet and more prone to back injuries, if you don't adjust to them.

Approximately two-thirds of women experience back pain in late pregnancy. This can be really tiring during the day, and makes sleeping difficult.

* Use pillows under your head or abdomen or behind your back to find a comfortable sleeping position.
* To get from lying down to standing, roll onto your side and push up with your arms. This prevents you placing extra strain on your back.
* Take care when lifting and twisting — you may not be able to lift or carry what you normally can.
* Try some regular low-impact exercise such as walking, aquarobics, hydrotherapy, pregnancy yoga or a Pilates class.
* Heat packs on the painful areas may also help, but it is important to talk to your healthcare provider beforehand as you want to be careful about raising your core body temperature.

Remember that if you are just starting any of the exercises above, see your healthcare provider first. If your back pain is becoming problematic it is important to talk to your healthcare provider as they may be able to refer you to a women's health physiotherapist for treatment.

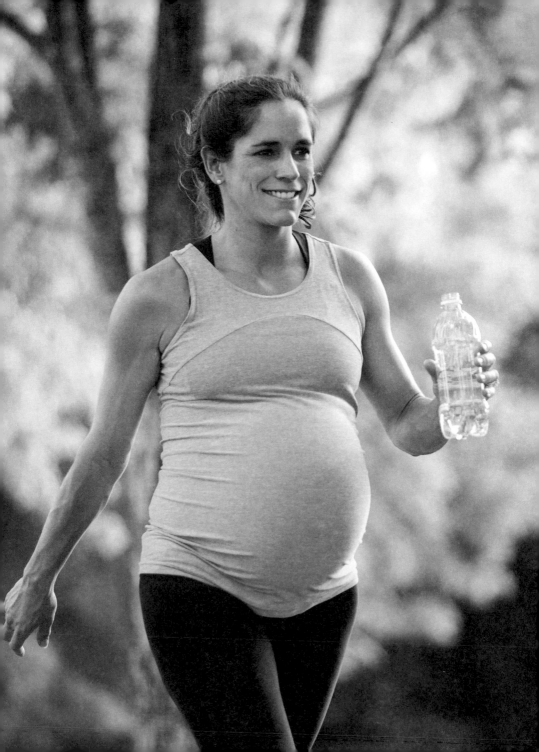

INDIGESTION/HEARTBURN/REFLUX

As mentioned in the first trimester section, indigestion or heartburn can occur more frequently as your pregnancy progresses. In the first trimester, indigestion is likely caused by increased levels of progesterone relaxing your muscles and slowing your digestion. But as you progress to the second and third trimesters your growing baby will increasingly push on the stomach and oesophageal sphincter (the ring of muscle between your stomach and throat). Together, the relaxed muscles and increased pressure can force food and stomach acids into your throat, causing that burning sensation. This can become worse when lying down, because you lose the help of gravity to keep the food and acids in your stomach.

* Eat smaller but more frequent meals during the day.
* Avoid large meals before bedtime.
* Limit spicy food and try eating and drinking at separate times.
* Sleep on your left-hand side to keep your stomach lower than your oesophagus.
* Elevate your head with pillows, or put foam wedges or rolled up towels under the top end of the mattress, to take some of the pressure off the oesophageal sphincter.

SWELLING

It is common and normal to have mild swelling in the face, hands, arms, legs and feet. This is because your body is producing approximately 50 per cent more blood and fluids, and also because your growing baby may be putting pressure on the veins carrying blood from your legs to your heart. You may discover that your rings or your shoes are harder to get on and off; or you may notice tingling and pressure in your feet and hands. This can be uncomfortable or painful and can disrupt your sleep.

It is important to talk to your healthcare provider if you have sudden or excessive swelling, swelling in only one hand/arm or foot/leg, constant headaches, vision changes, sensitivity to light, chest pains or difficulty breathing, as this can be a sign of pre-eclampsia.

Things you can do to help relieve the swelling:

* Try to stay cool.
* Avoid tight clothing around wrists and ankles.
* Rest with your feet elevated.
* Avoid standing for long periods of time.
* Use cold compresses on swollen areas.
* Ensure you are well hydrated.
* Try submerging your body in water (e.g. a pool or a bath with cool or warm water) to provide short-term relief.
* Frequently stretch your legs, flex or circle your hands and feet and wiggle your toes and fingers.
* Gentle, regular exercise will help with your circulation.
* Wear comfortable shoes.

CARPAL TUNNEL SYNDROME (CTS)

Swelling and fluid build-up around the bones and ligaments can crowd the small 'tunnel' in the wrist, which puts pressure on the nerve and tendons going from the forearm to the hand. If this occurs, you may feel symptoms such as tingling, numbness, weakness and pain in the fingers, thumb, hand and/or arm, which can make it difficult to find a comfortable sleeping position, or can wake you from your sleep. Fluid retention in the hands is more likely in the third trimester, and this may be why more women experience CTS at this stage of their pregnancy. If you are experiencing any of these symptoms, see your healthcare provider, who may be able to suggest ways to relieve the symptoms or refer you to a specialist.

RESTLESS LEGS SYNDROME

We mentioned RLS in the second trimester, but symptoms can become more common in the third trimester. Restless legs syndrome is the irresistible urge to move your legs, often accompanied by unpleasant sensations such as burning, itching or tingling. These sensations are usually stronger when your legs are still; for example, when you are trying to sleep. Sleep loss and stress are known to be contributors to RLS, as are low levels of iron and folate. Massage, relaxation and stretching can help relieve symptoms. Because caffeine limits the absorption of folate, limiting caffeine intake can also help.

LEG CRAMPS

Approximately 30 per cent of pregnant women experience leg cramps, most commonly in the second and third trimesters. Leg cramps are a painful contraction of the foot or calf muscle (or sometimes both). Even after the contraction releases, the pain can linger for around 10 minutes.

If you are suffering from leg cramps, the best treatment for immediate relief is flexing the foot to release the contraction. For persistent leg cramps, the most recent research has shown that vitamin B or magnesium supplements can help reduce or eliminate the cramps, but it's important to talk about this with your healthcare provider before you start taking any supplements. Although there is no research evidence to show that stretching before bedtime reduces leg cramps, anecdotal evidence suggests it's helpful. Quinine and vitamin E have been shown to have a positive effect on reducing leg cramps, but their use during pregnancy is not recommended.

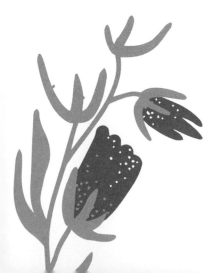

ANXIETY AND WORRY/INSOMNIA

As mentioned earlier, it is very common to have a busy mind when you hop into bed. In fact, nearly three-quarters of all pregnant women worry about their sleep in the third trimester or have some degree of insomnia. It is normal to have anxious thoughts about the health of your baby, the labour and/or delivery, finances or relationships.

Try the following strategies:

* Keep a notepad and pencil next to your bed and write your thoughts down. You can always return to those thoughts if need be in the morning.
* Talking about your fears or worries can help process your thoughts and reduce stress and anxiety. Try chatting with your partner, family member, friend or a professional who is able to listen and help.
* Use music or relaxation/meditation strategies or apps to help calm the mind before sleep.
* Try a gentle activity during the day — swimming, walking, aquarobics or yoga can all help improve your sleep.
* Mental imagery techniques like the one opposite can help calm a busy mind before sleep.
* The Australian Sleep Health Foundation website has information and strategies for helping insomnia — see www.sleephealthfoundation.org.au/insomnia.

It's important to talk to your healthcare provider if any of these worries or anxieties are causing you any distress.

**Try distracting your busy thoughts.
Focus on an image and concentrate
on the details . . .**

♡

Where are
you and what is
going on
around you?

♡

Are things
moving and
can you
follow that
movement?

♡

What can
you touch?
What is the
texture, shape
and size?

**Choose a joyful
and peaceful place
or event, somewhere
that makes you feel
happy, safe and relaxed.
This might be a room
in your house, the beach,
a park or a place
you've visited
on holiday.**

♡

What can
you taste?
Can you
taste food
or the air
around you?

♡

Why does
this place
feel so
relaxing?

♡

What can
you smell?
Is there just one
smell or lots
of different
ones?

♡

What is the
temperature of the
air and the things
around you?

♡

Who are
you with and
how do they make
you feel?

TIME TO GET UP

Not being able to switch off your thoughts can be very frustrating when you are feeling so exhausted. Remember, if you can't get to sleep within 20–30 minutes, get up and go to another room. This is very important, because you want your bedroom environment to invoke feelings of sleepiness and relaxation.

* Find a quiet, warm, low-light place in another room (such as a cosy chair in the lounge).
* Take your time doing something quiet (reading, craft, but not watching television or checking your mobile phone).
* When you start to feel sleepy again, try going back to bed.

DREAMS

As we said in the first trimester section, vivid dreams and nightmares are very common in pregnancy: 70 per cent of women experience them at some stage during their pregnancy. You are processing an enormous amount of change in a short period of time, and it's totally normal to feel overwhelmed, anxious, irritable or worried at the thought of being a new mother. Remember: dreams are not premonitions, they are just your brain's way of processing information. If nightmares or dreams are causing you distress, it might be helpful to talk about any worries or concerns with a partner, friend or your healthcare provider.

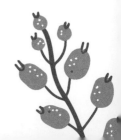

Other strategies for dealing with sleep and fatigue

In the third trimester you may be spending more time in the lighter stages of sleep and, if so, you will awaken more easily. Try a white noise app if noises such as snoring, barking or vehicles are waking you at night. White noise works by reducing the difference between loud sounds and background noise.

Use the 'downtime' function on your phone to silence notifications while you sleep. Downtime also provides reminders about when downtime is approaching, which may be helpful for starting your bedtime routine.

Is summer approaching? Consider investing in blackout curtains or blinds to keep the sunlight out of your bedroom in the late evenings, early mornings or when you are trying to nap.

Try not to fall asleep on the couch in the evenings. This reduces your brain's drive for sleep and can make it harder to fall asleep when you do go to bed.

If you have older toddlers or children, see if a friend or family member can help with childcare while you have some rest time.

Is your partner an 'owl' or 'lark', and is that different to you? Does this affect your bedtime or wake time because they are coming to bed late or waking early in the morning? Perhaps you or your partner could sleep in another bed on days when this occurs to make the most of your sleep opportunity.

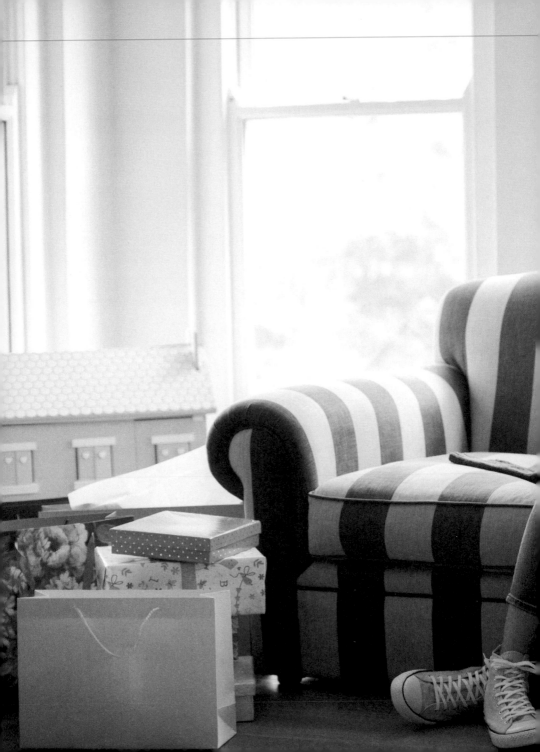

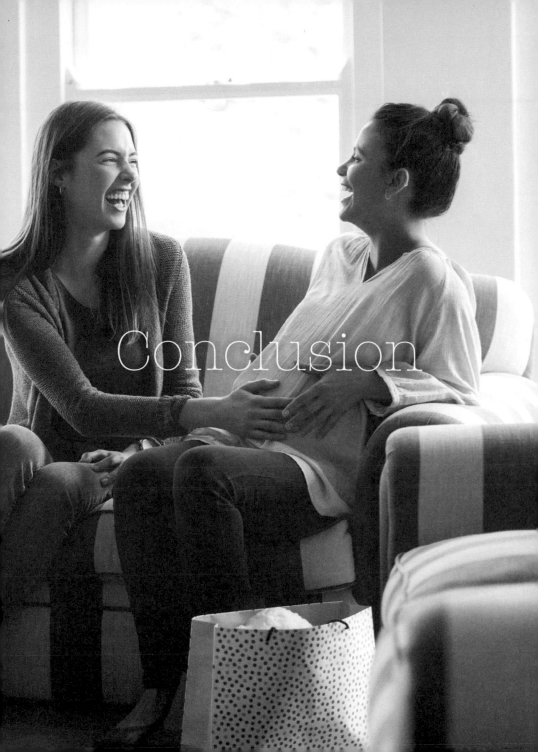

Conclusion

She used to say
she could taste sleep
and that it was as
delicious as a BLT on
fresh French bread.

— REBECCA WELLS, DIVINE SECRETS
OF THE YA-YA SISTERHOOD

This book came into existence because of a research study completed in 2017–18. We wanted to see if increasing women's sleep knowledge and normalising the sleep changes experienced in pregnancy could help improve women's moods. The study involved a small but amazing group of women who were provided with the information contained in this book. Even though the study needs to be repeated with a larger group of women, we noticed some interesting initial findings. Women really enjoyed learning about sleep; they understood their own sleep better and they felt reassured when they learnt why their sleep was changing. Importantly, their mood remained positive throughout. This wasn't completely unexpected, because there is now a large body of research that links sleep with both physical and mental health. Making the most of your sleep opportunities and limiting sleep disruptions can help improve your wellbeing — and your baby's wellbeing, too.

But we also understand the challenge of pregnancy sleep. Just when you need and want a good night's sleep, it feels completely unattainable! Please know, that's okay. Some nights will be great, other nights just okay and some nights will be tricky, even if you've tried every available strategy. Your body and mind are going through enormous change, so having the same sleep as before you were pregnant can be difficult at times. Be gentle on yourself. Rest when you can. Ask for help when you need it.

Whether you've read this book in one sitting or read it in parts as the different trimesters roll around, our message is the same. We wish you the very best for the months and years to come. Pregnancy, the birth, the initial few months with your little one, and the years beyond will be full of surprises. Yes, there will be challenges and rough patches, but there are also moments of pure happiness that will take your breath away. Again, be gentle on yourself. Rest when you can. Ask for help when you need it.

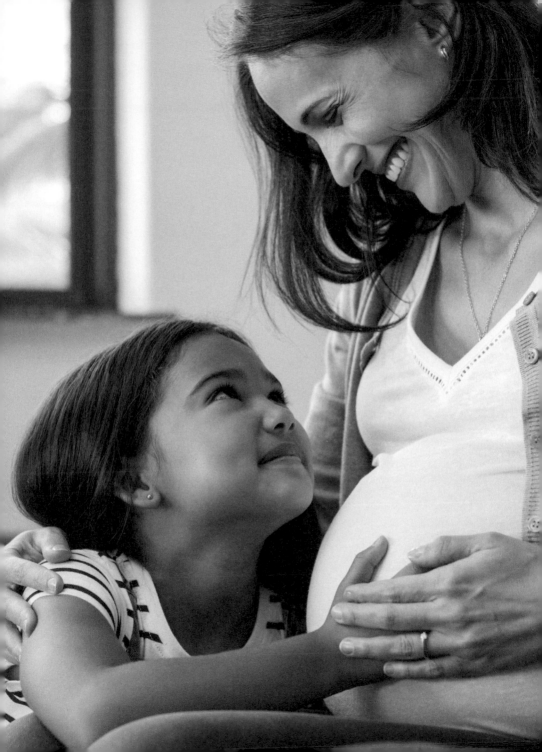

About the authors

'I could cope so much better if I could just get a good night's sleep.' This regularly repeated phrase from friends and mothers far and wide (as well as herself) is what prompted Clare Ladyman into the field of sleep science. Clare's PhD looked at how sleep and mental health are related throughout the pregnancy and postnatal periods, and how providing information on sleep can help reduce the likelihood of mothers experiencing depression. She completed her research studies at the Sleep/Wake Research Centre, Massey University, Wellington, and now lives in Perth, Western Australia, with her husband and two teenage boys (who finally now sleep . . . a lot).

Leigh Signal has been a sleep scientist for over 20 years. She is associate professor and portfolio director, Fatigue Management and Sleep Health, at the Sleep/Wake Research Centre, Massey University, Wellington. Ten years ago, when she was pregnant with her second child and struggling with her own sleep, she began a series of projects looking at the links between perinatal sleep and mothers' health. One of the projects she co-led was entitled E, Moe Māmā ('Go to sleep, mother'). Although when translated it sounds like an instruction, the name is meant to convey care, support and encouragement for mothers to be able to sleep well, which is what she hopes this book helps you do.

Clare and Leigh would like to thank Dr Bronwyn Sweeney, Professor Kathryn Lee, Dr Michel Sangalli and Dr Simon McDowell for their contributions to the making of this book.

About the Sleep/Wake Research Centre

A Health Research Council Repatriation Fellowship enabled Philippa Gander to return to New Zealand and establish the Sleep/Wake Research Centre in 1998 at Otago University School of Medicine, Wellington. In 2003 the Centre moved to Massey University, where it has thrived. The Centre is externally funded and is New Zealand's first laboratory dedicated to research and education in circadian physiology, sleep science and their applications.

The original three-bed time isolation unit at Massey was basic but adequate for sleep inertia and constant routine protocols, as well as some fascinating arts/science collaborative experiments. After the strong 2013 Wellington earthquake the building on Adelaide Road was found to be earthquake-prone and the Sleep/Wake Research Centre's long-awaited move to better premises was initiated. The new purpose-built premises on the top floor of Block 4 on Tasman Street, Mount Cook, are superb, with interior design by Ian Athfield Architects, and a new world-class four-bed time isolation facility.

The Centre focuses on three core areas:

Research

A central construct is that improving health, safety, productivity and wellbeing requires better understanding of the interactions between sleep and waking function, and their regulation by the circadian body clock. Our work in this shared discipline space is greatly enriched by the diverse disciplinary, professional and cultural backgrounds of our staff, students and collaborators.

Education

The Centre hosts and provides supervision for dedicated candidates at the master's, doctoral and postdoctoral level. We offer undergraduate and postgraduate university courses, as well as lectures, seminars and workshops for a diverse range of groups and organisations.

Consulting

Centre staff have broad experience in evidence-based consulting for government agencies, industries and unions in the areas of shift work and fatigue management. We also have broad experience in independent accident investigation and expert testimony relating to these areas.

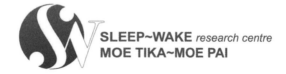

SLEEP~WAKE *research centre*
MOE TIKA~MOE PAI

Index

Numbers in **bold** indicate diagrams